ICE HOCKEY SHORT STORIES FOR KIDS

Charlotte Gibbs

© Copyright 2023 - All rights reserved.

The content contained within this book may not be reproduced, duplicated or transmitted without direct written permission from the author or the publisher.

Under no circumstances will any blame or legal responsibility be held against the publisher, or author, for any damages, reparation, or monetary loss due to the information contained within this book, either directly or indirectly.

Legal Notice:

This book is copyright protected. It is only for personal use. You cannot amend, distribute, sell, use, quote or paraphrase any part, or the content within this book, without the consent of the author or publisher.

Disclaimer Notice:

Please note the information contained within this document is for educational and entertainment purposes only. All effort has been executed to present accurate, up to date, reliable, complete information. No warranties of any kind are declared or implied. Readers acknowledge that the author is not engaged in the rendering of legal, financial, medical or professional advice. The content within this book has been derived from various sources. Please consult a licensed professional before attempting any techniques outlined in this book.

By reading this document, the reader agrees that under no circumstances is the author responsible for any losses, direct or indirect, that are incurred as a result of the use of the information contained within this document, including, but not limited to, errors, omissions, or inaccuracies.

TABLE OF CONTENTS

Introduction
6

CHAPTER 1
Magnificent Mario
8

CHAPTER 2
Gumper Never Gives Up
13

CHAPTER 3
The Greatest Game Nobody Saw
18

CHAPTER 4
The Miracle on Ice
23

CHAPTER 5
Brothers and Sisters
28

CHAPTER 6
The Dawson City Nuggets
34

CHAPTER 7
Calling All Goalies
39

CHAPTER 8
Breaking Barriers
44

CHAPTER 9
Tales of the Stanley Cup
49

CHAPTER 10
Batman
54

CHAPTER 11
Meeting Your Idol
59

CHAPTER 12
The Rocket Nets Five - Twice!
63

CHAPTER 13
Geared Up
67

CHAPTER 14
Upset
72

CHAPTER 15
Tootoo
77

CHAPTER 16
Number Four, Bobby Orr
83

CHAPTER 17
It's Okay Not to be Okay
88

CHAPTER 18
Baun Scores On One Leg
92

CHAPTER 19
Adjust Your Vision
96

CHAPTER 20
The Merry Prankster
100

Conclusion
105

INTRODUCTION

We all face difficult times, right? Maybe there's a subject at school you struggle with, or perhaps you think you're too young to start chasing your dreams. Well, this is where *Ice Hockey Short Stories* for Kids steps in. In these short stories, you'll meet a collection of brave athletes, read about their inspiring stories, and, hopefully, learn something valuable.

Even the most prominent athletes in the world struggle sometimes and are constantly defying the odds to prove themselves. From hilarious nicknames and pranks to very real stories about mental health and physical setbacks, there's a little piece of inspiration here for everyone.

The history of ice hockey dates back to 1875, when the first official game was played in Montreal, Canada. I mean, of course, it started out in Canada, right? It was influenced by a combination of 18th-century sports, such as lacrosse and hurling. Would you believe that some of the original rules and field markings are still present to this day? These stories span across the long history of ice hockey, showing us that these funny mishaps or tough challenges have been present for years and years.

Whether you're here to just learn a little more about the stories behind your favorite sport or you want to learn some valuable lessons, let's get reading! So, lace up your skates, grab your hockey stick, and get ready for a thrilling adventure of inspirational tales.

CHAPTER 1

MAGNIFICENT MARIO

Ever since he was a young boy playing hockey in Verdun, Quebec, Mario Lemieux was seen as a player who was destined for greatness. By the time he was in his last year of Junior hockey, there was little doubt Mario would be the first player chosen in the 1984 NHL Draft. In 70 games, he scored an astounding 133 goals and 149 assists for a whopping total of 282 points. Knowing they couldn't miss out on the opportunity to acquire a player like Lemieux, the Pittsburgh Penguins made it their mission to finish dead last in the NHL so they could draft Lemieux, which they did.

When he stepped onto the ice for his first game in a Pittsburgh uniform, excited Penguin fans were in for a treat. On his first shift against the Boston Bruins, Lemieux would score the first goal of his career. Suddenly, hockey in Pittsburgh was exciting again, even if it wasn't seen in the standings. Mario would win the Calder Trophy as the league's outstanding rookie. It wasn't too long before he earned the nickname Magnificent Mario. Soon, a ticket to a Penguins game became like gold, and fans flocked to see a player who was challenging Wayne Gretzky as the best player in the world. By 1991, he would lead the Penguins to their first Stanley Cup, a feat they would repeat the following season.

When the 1992-93 season started, the Penguins looked ready to make it three Stanley Cups in a row. Lemieux was at the top of the league in scoring, setting a record by scoring at least one goal in 12 straight games. Even Gretzky's records of 92 goals and 215 points in one season looked like they might be in jeopardy of falling. Then, Lemieux shocked the world.

In early January of 1993, at a tearful press conference, Mario announced he had cancer and that he would be starting treatment right away. He was quitting hockey to try and get better. Fans and teammates wanted the best for their hero but wondered if he'd ever again play the game he loved so much. If he did come back, it wouldn't be that season. But Mario never backed down from a challenge. He was going to beat the disease, so he started a vigorous treatment process that would cause him to miss two months of the season. Getting healthy was the most important factor, not playing hockey. And everyone across the league, no matter who they played for, was rooting for Mario.

Then, a surprise. On March 2, 1993, Mario received his last treatment, boarded a plane, and joined the Penguins in Philadelphia. That night, the Penguins were preparing to play their bitter rivals, the Philadelphia Flyers. Even his teammates didn't know he was coming, so when he joined them in the locker room, it was a pleasant surprise for everyone. As Mario skated onto the Philadelphia ice, the usually hostile Flyers fans gave him a standing ovation. When he started treatment, Lemieux found himself 12 points behind Buffalo's Pat Lafontaine with only 19 games remaining. In his first game back, he scored. He would win the scoring title by 12 points with 160 points in 60 games.

That story alone would be enough to solidify Lemieux's place in hockey history, but there is more. In 1997, Mario once again decided he had to leave hockey. His back had been failing him for years, and the pain was too much. But he didn't stay away from the Penguins for long, eventually buying the Penguins franchise, saving it from possibly moving from Pittsburgh. He also never lost his passion to be a player. So, after four years away, he decided he'd sign himself and once again become a player. He'd be the only modern team owner to also be a player.

From the sidelines, the game looked easy for Mario Lemieux, and in some ways, it was. But when something is easy, it is winning the hard battles that show what character someone has. Mario battled hard to bring the Penguins from one of the weakest teams in the league to one of the best and then conquered the personal health battles he faced as a player. He proved that no matter how tough things might seem, if you work hard, you can overcome all obstacles.

Lemieux teaches us that, with dedication and fighting battles, you are more than capable of overcoming challenges, and you'll come out strong. Facing obstacles and setbacks is part of being human, but it's what we do with those challenges and how we make a comeback that shows our true character.

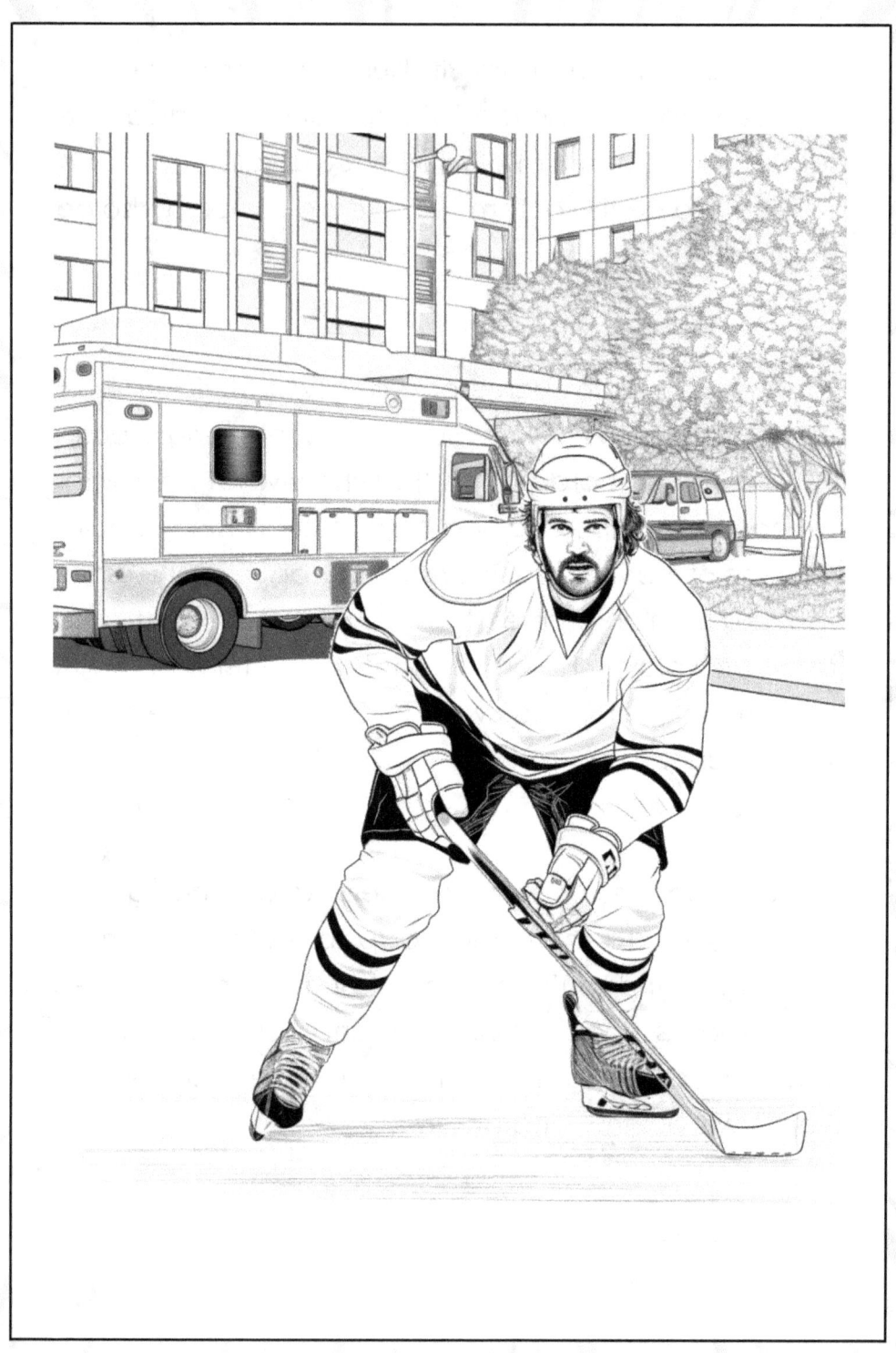

CHAPTER 2

GUMPER NEVER GIVES UP

When goaltender Lorne Worsley arrived at his first junior hockey camp, his team wanted to know if he had a nickname. He didn't have one, so as a joke, he wrote down the first thing that came to his mind: Gump. And with that legend of Gump Worsley was born. What funny nickname would you give yourself if you were put on the spot like that?

He wasn't the biggest kid; he stood only 5 feet, 7 inches, the average height of most ice hockey players is 6 feet, 1 inch, nor was he the most skilled. But he was a good athlete with a passion for ice hockey and a desire to win. Still, to make it to the NHL was tough—Worsley knew that not everyone made it to the league. There were only six teams, two goalies per team. With only 12 spots available, it was going to be hard to make it as a professional goalie.

But for the young Gump, he was determined to succeed, no matter the challenges.

After a successful career in junior hockey, Gump was soon signed by the New York Rangers and started playing in their minor league system as a goalie. He would start in New Haven, Connecticut, then bounced around the minor hockey world, going everywhere from St. Paul, Minnesota, to Saskatoon, Saskatchewan, then on to Vancouver, and back to Saskatoon. Finally, after four years, he got his shot as a rookie with the NHL's Rangers, who were the league's worst team at the time, but Gump didn't care about that–he was in! Despite being on a team that managed only 17 wins in a 70-game season, Gump was a standout goalie and would go on to win the Calder Trophy as the NHL's top rookie.

But when the next season rolled around, Gump was back in the minors, sent there after a salary dispute. He'd spend two more years in the minors before the Rangers realized their mistake and brought him back up. It was true; they really needed him. He'd be the mainstay on a team that was never very good. When asked what team gave Gump the most problems, the comedic Worsley joked 'The New York Rangers.'

Despite playing the next nine years in New York, Gump and the Rangers saw little success, with a second-place finish in 1957-58 being their best season. By 1963, the Rangers traded him to the Montreal Canadiens, who already had good goalies, so once again, Gump would find himself in the minors, this time in Quebec City. Still determined, he played like he deserved to go back to the NHL, and in the middle of the 1965 season, he was called up to the Canadiens. That spring, he would be in nets as the Canadiens would win the Stanley Cup, the first of Gump's career. For the next four years, he'd be a fixture in nets for the Canadiens, winning three more Stanley Cups and two Vezina Trophies as the league's top goalie. But by 1970, at 40 years of age, he decided he'd had enough. Where teams used to take road trips by train, they were now taking them by airplane, and Gump hated to fly, so he hung up his skates…at least for a while, that is.

Needing help in goal, the young Minnesota North Stars (now the Dallas Stars) lured him out of retirement, and he would go on to play four more years in the league. When he finally did retire for the last time at age 44, he'd won 335 games in the NHL, posted 48 shutouts, and finished with a Goals Against Average of 2.88, all done while never wearing a goalie's mask. In 1980, the goalie who seemed to be the player nobody wanted for a long time, being swapped between teams and handed off as if he were a nuisance to them, was elected to hockey's highest honor when he was made a member of the Hockey Hall of Fame.

So, what can we take from Gump's career? Gump Worsely's determination proved that you should never give up on your dream, never let anyone decide you're not good enough, and never believe it is too late to make a difference.

No matter how many people tell you you'll never make it or perhaps even poke fun at you for having an ambitious goal, remember that your dreams are valid, and you never know when your opportunity will come. Like Gump, never let go of that glimmer of hope; the world has a place for you, and you will get there.

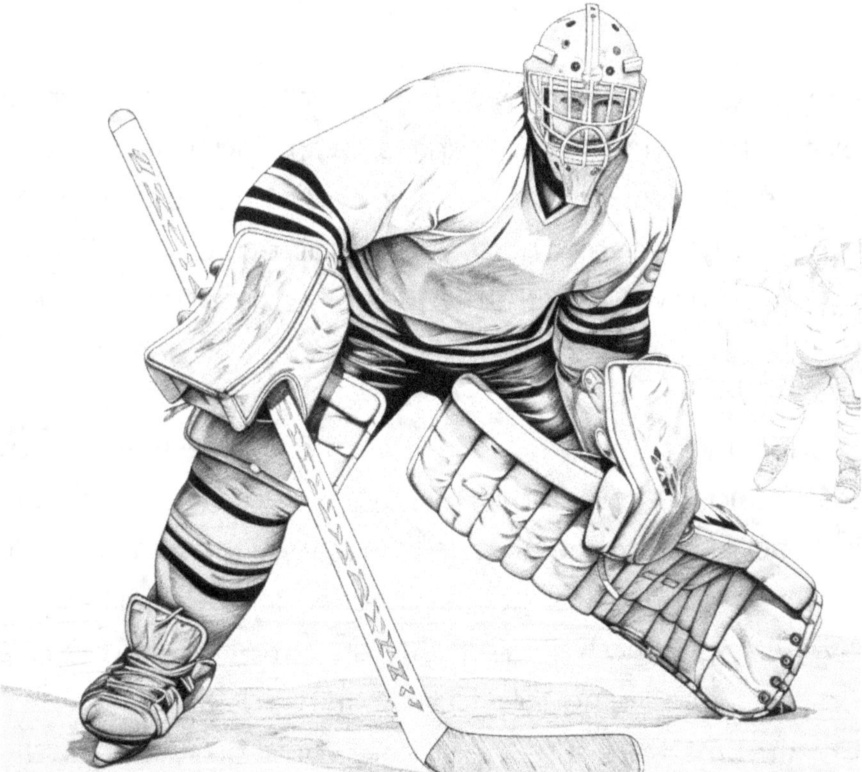

CHAPTER 3

THE GREATEST GAME NOBODY SAW

Everybody loves a snow day. You wake up; there's snow everywhere, and it is still falling, slowly piling up inches and inches of a thick blanket of snow. You turn on the TV or radio, maybe even check your email, eagerly waiting for the good news. And then you see it: school is canceled.

In January of 1987, that's just what both the New Jersey Devils and Calgary Flames thought would happen, except instead of school being canceled, they thought it would be their game. A huge snowstorm stopped just about everything in the New York City area that day, and since people were being told to stay off roads and highways, both teams were sure the game would be rescheduled.

Since Calgary were the visitors, they arrived early at the Brendan Byrne Arena together. Somehow, their bus managed to make the drive to the game. According to NHL rules, if the visitors show up, then the game has to be played. The Devils, on the other hand, were coming from all over New York and New Jersey, and by 7:30 p.m., when the game was supposed to start, they still didn't have enough players. The weather was delaying all of their arrivals, despite Calgary managing to arrive well on time from Canada. It wouldn't be until 9 p.m. that they were finally ready to play some hockey that evening.

But what about the fans? Under 12,000 tickets were sold for the game, and the majority of fans thought that the game would be canceled and stayed home—they, like both teams, believed the game would not go ahead. There were, however, a mere 334 diehard Devils' fans who made it to the arena that day; some, they say, arrived by snowmobile.

When the game eventually started, fans could hear the players talking on the ice, and the players could hear the fans in the stalls—that's how quiet and empty the arena was. In a normal game, there would be thousands of fans screaming, cheering, and shouting, and you'd never stand a chance of feeling so close to the players. One fan even interacted personally with the linesman after a questionable call. It was just that quiet in the cavernous, 19,000-seat arena. Imagine this: you go see a game, or maybe your favorite singer in concert, and bad weather means you're one of only 300 people to show up; it's so empty that you actually get to interact with them, and they can hear you! That's how these ice hockey fans felt that day.

The game's opening goal was scored by Perry Anderson, who wasn't even supposed to play that night. When some players couldn't make it, he was pressed into service on the rink. The game itself turned into a wild affair, with the Devils getting out to a 2-1 lead after the first period. They made it 3-1 early in the second, but the Flames stormed back with three straight goals to take a 4-3 lead. The third period was all New Jersey as they would score four goals to Calgary's one to win the game 7-5. The back-and-forth game thrilled the fans who were there and even the arena staff, who could be seen watching from the entrances due to the lack of business at the concessions.

For those fans who showed up, they would not be forgotten. During the game, representatives of the Devil's organization took down every fan's name and address. A few weeks later, every fan who was at the game received a letter from the Devil's organization and a special pin, making them official members of the "334 Club". To this day, it still ranks as the lowest-attended game in the history of the NHL.

Those ice hockey fans, like both teams, persevered despite the weather and showed up to support them. This game shows us that if you are continuously showing up for something or someone, you will eventually see the rewards and be recognized for your dedication.

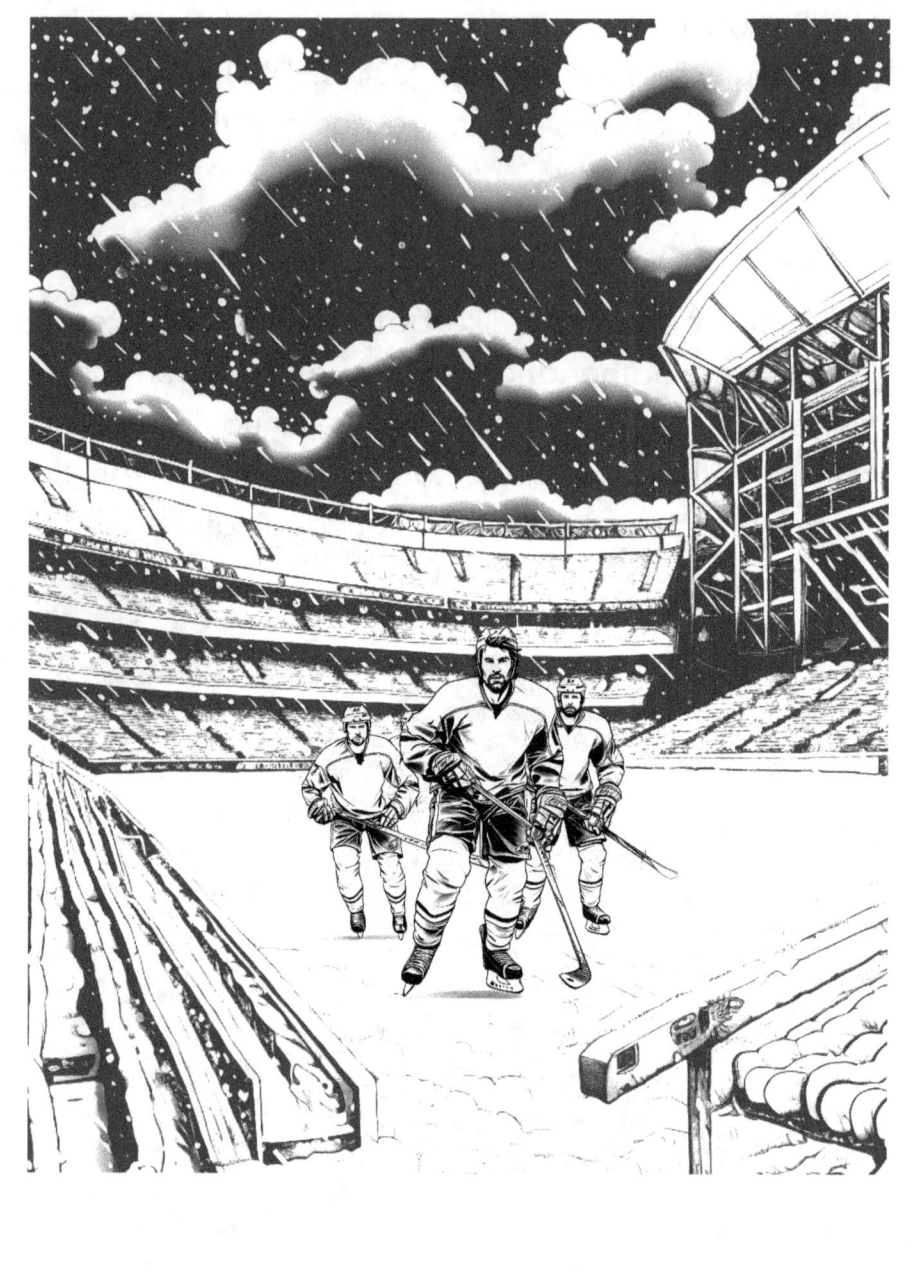

CHAPTER 4

THE MIRACLE ON ICE

When the 1980 Winter Olympics were awarded to Lake Placid, New York, there was a worry that interest in the Winter Games was fading. Lake Placid had hosted the games before in 1932, but when they won the bid for 1980, it was because all other candidates to host withdrew due to lack of funds or interest. I guess you could say they were pretty much the last resort.

As the games approached, interest started to grow as many American athletes were considered favorites to win gold in their events. One team that wasn't given much, if any, consideration was the US Men's Hockey Team. At the time, only amateur athletes could compete in the Olympics, which meant Team USA would be made up of college players.

The same went for other national teams, except for Russia, then known as the Union of Soviet Socialist Republics or the USSR. Their players were considered amateurs even though they all played in Russia's top league. Since they were all part of the Russian Army, they were considered soldiers and, therefore, amateurs. But they didn't play like amateurs.

There was no doubt the Russians were the tournament favorites. They'd won two consecutive World Championships, 13 of the last 16 and the last four Olympic golds. They were led by goalie Vladislav Tretiak, who would go on to be the first player trained outside of North America to be elected to the Hockey Hall of Fame. The year before, they beat a team made up of NHL All-Stars two games to one in a best-of-three series. You can clearly see they are certainly not amateurs.

On the other hand, the Americans were a hodge-podge of college players who were thrown together and not given much hope. Unlike today, college hockey, while good, wasn't up to the standards of the NHL and certainly as good as an international powerhouse like the Russians. If there were any further doubt, this would be a tough tournament for the Americans to even get a medal, let alone win; they would lose their last exhibition game before the Olympics 10-3 to the Russians in New York.

The good news for the USA was they would not have to face the Russians in the preliminary round. They opened with a surprising 2-2 tie with Sweden and then stunned Czechoslovakia with a 7-3 win. This meant the Americans had a place in the medal round, and their coach, Herb Brooks, was convinced they had a chance. With a packed house in the tiny Olympic arena, the college kids were determined to show that the exhibition game was a fluke and that they were just as good as the other teams.

And now, it was time for the American team to play against Russia. With the eyes of the world watching, the Americans fell behind 1-0, and fans were slowly losing hope. With six minutes to go in the first period, they would bring the game to a tie. In the last few minutes, the Russians would retake the lead, but the feisty and determined Americans scored in the last second for a 2-2 tie. The Russians would score the only goal of period two, but the Americans were feeling good about themselves being down only one goal heading into the third.

The Americans came after the Russians, and midway through the period, forward Mark Johnson would tie the game at 3-3. Mere minutes later, USA captain Mike Eruzione would give his team the lead, one which they held onto until the very end. As the final seconds ticked down, broadcaster Al Michaels uttered his famous call: "Do you believe in miracles? YES!" The USA would, you guessed it, end up winning this game against Russia.

Two days later, USA would go on to beat Finland in their final game and win the gold, forever solidifying the team as a powerhouse in hockey history.

So, what can we take from the USA team's incredible miracle? You may have people doubting your abilities or perhaps some intimidating upcoming challenges, but perseverance is the best way to prove people wrong and overcome them. Like this hockey team, even when things feel they may be going downhill, there is always a little miraculous way to come out stronger than ever and make history.

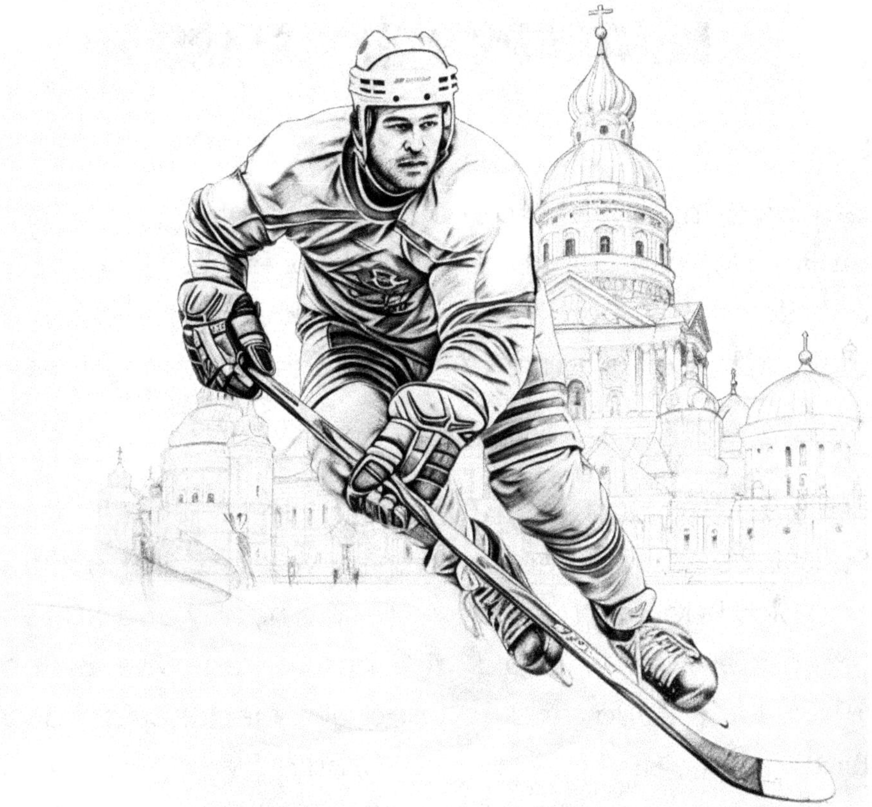

CHAPTER 5

BROTHERS AND SISTERS

Getting to the NHL is hard enough as it is, but when brothers make it together, it is even more impressive. Many pairs of brothers have made it to the big leagues, and some of them became important parts of their team victories.

Early in the 20th Century, outside of Saskatoon, Saskatchewan, the Bentley brothers were learning to skate and play hockey–they enjoyed it as a hobby and started to wonder where it could take them career-wise. By the 1940s, Max, Doug, and Reg had all joined the Chicago Blackhawks, and in 1943, they would form the first line made up entirely of brothers. Max and Doug would go on to be elected to the Hockey Hall of Fame. What was once a simple shared passion between brothers became a viable career and changed their lives forever. Who knows if they could've done it without each other?

In Montreal, Maurice 'The Rocket' Richard, a player for the Montreal Canadiens, had established himself as one of the best players in the game. In 1945, he became the first player in league history to score 50 goals in a season, achieving it in just 50 games–what an impressive achievement! In 1955, his brother Henri followed in Maurice's footsteps and joined the Canadiens, and together, they would win five straight Stanley Cups. Henri earned himself the nickname 'Pocket Rocket', a hilarious nod to his brother's nickname. When Maurice retired in 1960, he'd scored a whopping 544 goals for his team, a record for the Canadiens that still stands to this day. Not to be outdone, Henri holds a record that will likely never be broken: he won an impressive total of 11 Stanley Cups as an ice hockey player.

In the little town of Viking, Alberta, summers are for farming, winters for playing hockey. Life was full of simplicities, and many kids in Viking played hockey for fun, but no one took it as seriously as the six Sutter brothers. Yes, you read that right, six of them! All six would not only play junior hockey, but they would all be drafted into the NHL. Brian would play his entire career with the St. Louis Blues, Darryl was with Chicago, Duane would go to the New York Islanders and win two Stanley Cups along with brother Brent, and twins Rich and Ron would go to rivals Philadelphia and Pittsburgh, respectively. How incredible is that? Brian,

Darryl, and Duane would also go on to coach in the NHL, and Darryl would win the Stanley Cup as coach of the Los Angeles Kings.

Back in Chicago, Dennis and Bobby Hull would transform the Blackhawks into Stanley Cup Champions by filling the net with puck after puck. They would score a huge total of 913 NHL goals between them. Bobby's son Brett would also play in the NHL, scoring 741 goals of his own between 1986 and 2005. Together, they hold the record for most goals scored by one family.

The record for most points by a set of brothers belongs, not surprisingly, to the Gretzky brothers, Wayne and Keith. Between them, they scored 2,861 points in the NHL, 2,857 by Wayne and four by Keith. Hey, a record is a record!

And last, what about sisters? Well, when Cammi Granato was growing up, she'd follow brothers Tony and Don to the ice rinks around Downers Grove, Illinois. While her big brothers would both make the NHL, Tony as a player and Don as a coach, Cammi would achieve something even better. She would win Olympic Gold and Silver medals while playing for Team USA at the 1996 and 2000 Olympic

Games. And she did make the NHL, just with a slightly different route, as the assistant General Manager with the Vancouver Canucks.

These sibling teams teach us that there's great power in family and that if you surround yourself with like-minded people, you can go on to achieve great things. Maybe you and your sibling dream of becoming pro athletes, or you and your bestie want to start a business together. Whatever it is, you can achieve a lot with close people by your side.

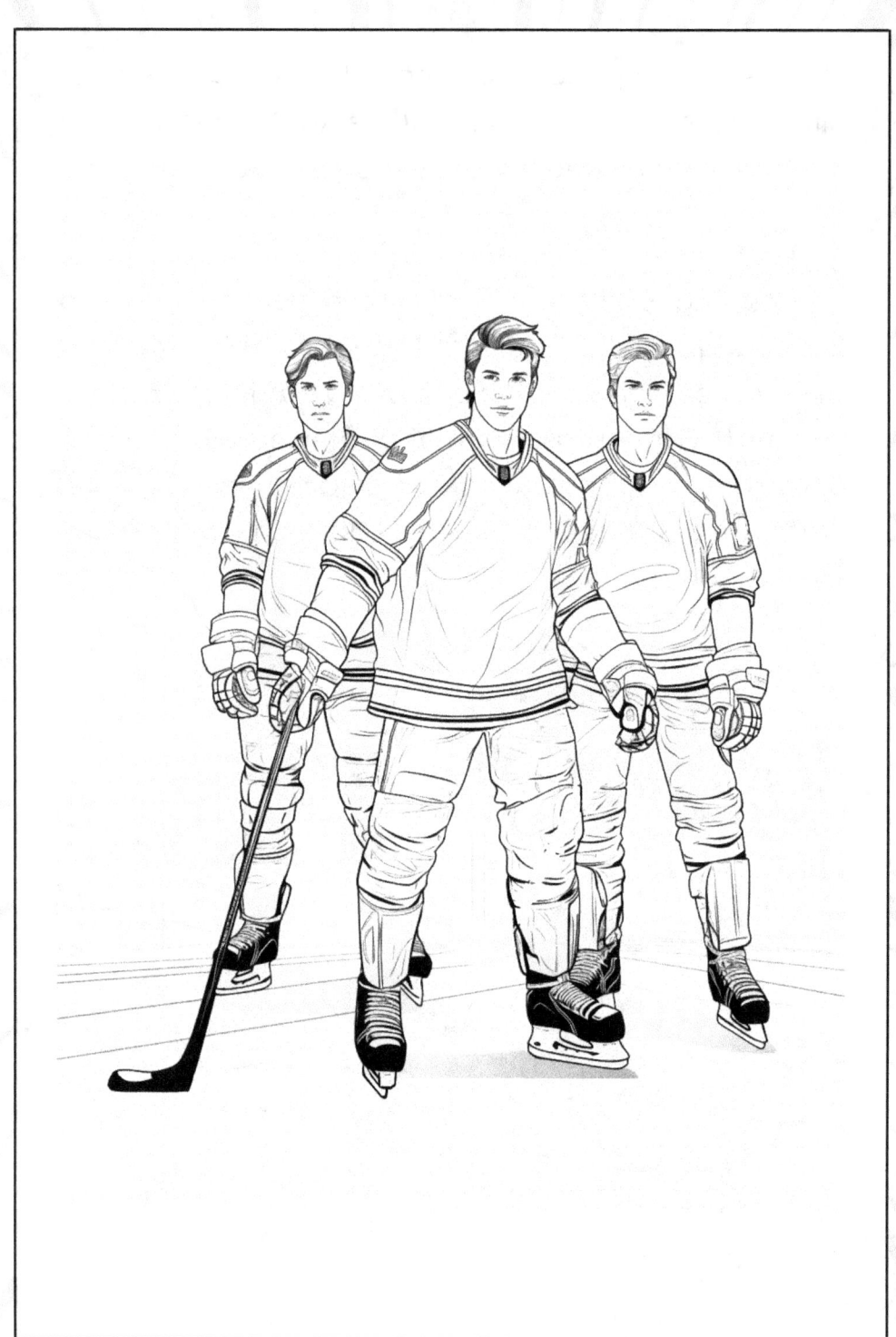

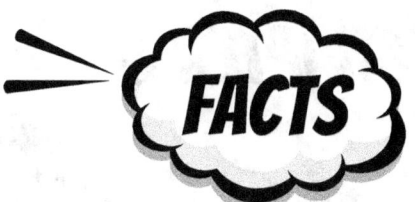

1. Ice hockey began in Canada in the early 1800s and swiftly spread to other cold-weather areas.

2. Due to the rapid pace at which players travel on the rink, hockey is frequently considered to be the fastest game on the planet.

3. A hat trick is when players score 3 goals in a game. To celebrate, fans traditionally throw their hats onto the ice.

4. When fired, A professional ice hockey puck can travel 100 miles per hour.

5. Many hockey players have superstitions concerning how they tape their sticks. Some people believe it brings good fortune and improves performance on the ice.

CHAPTER 6

THE DAWSON CITY NUGGETS

Did you know before the National Hockey League took possession of the Stanley Cup, any team in Canada could challenge for the trophy? It is true. No matter how big or small, any team could snatch this trophy.

Donated by Governor General Lord Stanley of Preston in 1893, the original cup was the bowl that sits atop the trophy (the modern version is a replica) and cost about $50 to make. It was originally intended for amateur teams alone, and any team could challenge the cup holders. In the early years, the cup changed hands several times as teams were eager to take their shot at winning the prize–everyone was desperate for a chance to win.

By 1905, the cup had been awarded to many different teams, but all of them came from either Ottawa, Montreal, or Winnipeg. But a challenge was brewing from a part of Canada that was far away from the hearts and minds of hockey fans of the day - little low-populated Dawson City.

In Dawson City, Yukon, the Dawson City Nuggets thought they had what it took to win the cup and wrestle it from the hands of teams in Canada's biggest cities–what big ambitions they had! The Ottawa Silver Seven, also known as the Senators, were the current cup holders and considered the best team in Canada and, therefore, the world. They were led by Frank 'One Eyed' McGee, who would score 135 goals in only 45 games over his four seasons with Ottawa.

Dawson's team was made up of men who worked in mining camps. Only two of their players had elite hockey experience. Weldon Young had played for Ottawa several years before, and Randy McLennan played on a team that challenged the Montreal Victorias in 1895. Despite the talent gap, the Nuggets had the financial backing, and with the challenge accepted, the team was ready to make the trip to Ottawa.

Dawson City was kind of in the middle of nowhere, and so the long commute began. Some players set out by dog sled, others by bicycle, and then the whole team got on a boat. Along the way, many players experienced seasickness. Fog forced the team to bypass Vancouver and head to Seattle, meaning they were delayed and missed their train to Ottawa. They were two days away from game one of the series when they finally arrived. Even worse, Young, their best player, still hadn't arrived, and Ottawa would not change the dates of the game.

Fatigue and the fact that Ottawa was the better team would be the difference. Dawson would lose game one 9-2 despite being down a respectable 3-1 at the half. Game two was even worse, as Ottawa would score 23 goals — 14 by McGee alone — for a 23-2 win. The game remains the most lopsided Stanley Cup score of all time.

Despite the loss, Dawson remains the smallest city to ever play for the Stanley Cup, and their story will forever be part of the trophy's lore. Even though they didn't win, they made history and defied the odds, and isn't that a win in itself?

So, what do we do when we fight so hard to win like the Dawson's did but still lose? It's important to remember that not every win means winning a trophy, coming out on top, or getting exactly what we want. There are lessons in losing that teach us valuable things and help us prosper in other ways, and that's a win, too!

Maybe your team loses a game, but you've learned how to play better next time. Perhaps you didn't get the grade you wanted, but now you know where you need to improve next time. The Dawson City Nuggets didn't win this game (even though they did make history), but they will have learned a lot about themselves and how to improve in future games.

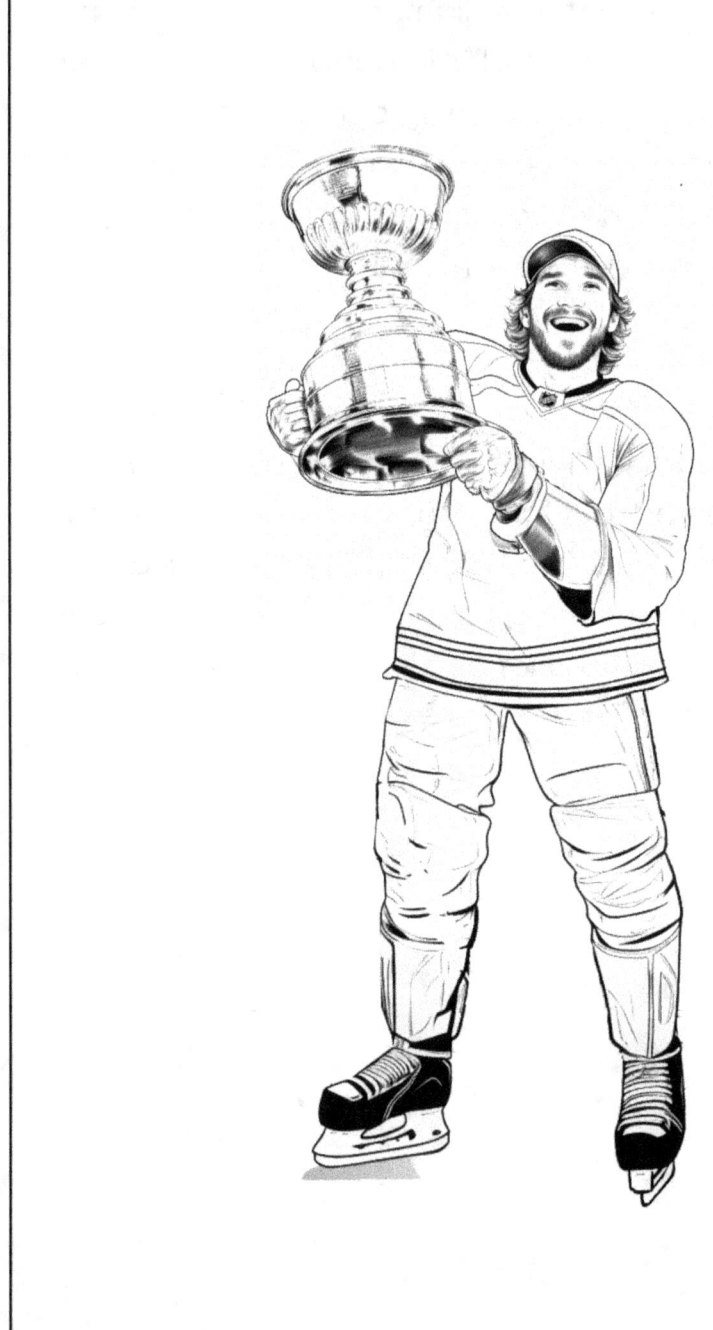

CHAPTER 7

CALLING ALL GOALIES

It is hard to argue that the most important player on a team is your goalie. But what happens if your goalie gets injured and then your backup goalie has a similar fate? Well, there are at least two examples of this happening in the National Hockey League, and both times, the results were a surprise.

The first time was back in 1928. The New York Rangers, who had only been a team for two years, were in the Stanley Cup final against the Montreal Maroons (Montreal had two NHL teams in those days). Rangers' goalie Lorne Chabot was hit in the eye with a shot and forced to leave the game. The Rangers had no backup goalie (it was not uncommon then), and Montreal refused a request by the Rangers to use Ottawa Senators goalie Alex Connell, who was at the game.

With no other options, the Rangers General Manager Lester Patrick, who was 44 at the time, went to the dressing room at the Montreal Forum and put on the goalie's pads. Imagine that! You're a manager standing on the sides, and now, all of a sudden, you're getting ready to go onto the rink. Anything for your team, right? The game was tied 0-0 when Patrick took over. With his team focusing on defense, he let in only one goal, and the result was a 1-1 at the end of regulation. Heading into overtime, the Maroons poured it on, but Patrick held the fort, and the Rangers would win when Frank Boucher scored. The Rangers would win their first Stanley Cup that day because of their GM.

More recently, in 2020, it would be the Carolina Hurricanes who would look to the stands for help. Playing the Maple Leafs in Toronto, Carolina would first lose starting goalie James Reimer in the first period, then backup Petr Mrazek midway through the second period. Two goalies down in one game, and things weren't looking good. Today, all NHL teams are required to have an emergency goalie on hand in case a team loses both backstops, and Carolina's misfortune meant 42-year-old David Ayres, a Zamboni driver who would often substitute at Carolina practices, was sent in—would he be able to save this game for Carolina?

Have you ever seen a Zamboni? They are those vehicles that drive around the rink and resurface the ice, making a smooth surface for ice hockey players, or even ice skaters, to use. So, there Ayres was - used to just driving his Zamboni around, but now he's on the rink in skates in hopes of helping lead the Carolina Hurricanes to victory.

Anyways, enough Zamboni talk. Down 3-1, the Maple Leafs saw this as an opportunity to get back into and win the game. Perhaps a substitution could rewrite this game. Nervous (I mean, wouldn't you be?), Ayres would give up two goals after coming in, but 'his' Hurricanes were still leading 4-3 with 20 minutes to go. In the third, Ayres would shut out his hometown Leafs, leading to a 6-3 Carolina win. The Zamboni-driving substitution turned out to be the best choice Carolina could've made that day. Ayres took this responsibility in his stride and proved a great asset to the team.

Ayres' lone NHL game would be news around the world, and he was recognized by politicians and fans. His number 90 jersey was sold with proceeds going to charity, he was made an honorary citizen of North Carolina, and the stick he used in the game was sent for display at the Hockey Hall of Fame.

There are two lessons we can use from this goalie substitute fiasco. Firstly, imagine being Ayres. You're a Zamboni driver whose sole job is to resurface and smoothen out the ice rink before, after, and mid-game. You'd never think that a team would lose enough backups for you to step in, but there you are. The pressure is on, and you don't let yourself crumble. So, what do we do when suddenly faced with a new, perhaps unexpected, responsibility? Take a page from Ayres' book and take it in your stride. Make the best of a tricky situation and do the best job you can.

Secondly, Ayres shows us that being nervous is okay, and frankly quite normal. Nerves are part of our human nature. Everyone feels nervous, even the biggest stars in the world before they step on stage. Ayres managed to get his nerves under control and used them to drive himself forward. So, how can we control our nerves? Have a little think about what makes you feel relaxed. Maybe listening to your favorite song or talking to close friends. Whatever it is, accept that it's okay to be nervous, and there are plenty of ways to learn to control them.

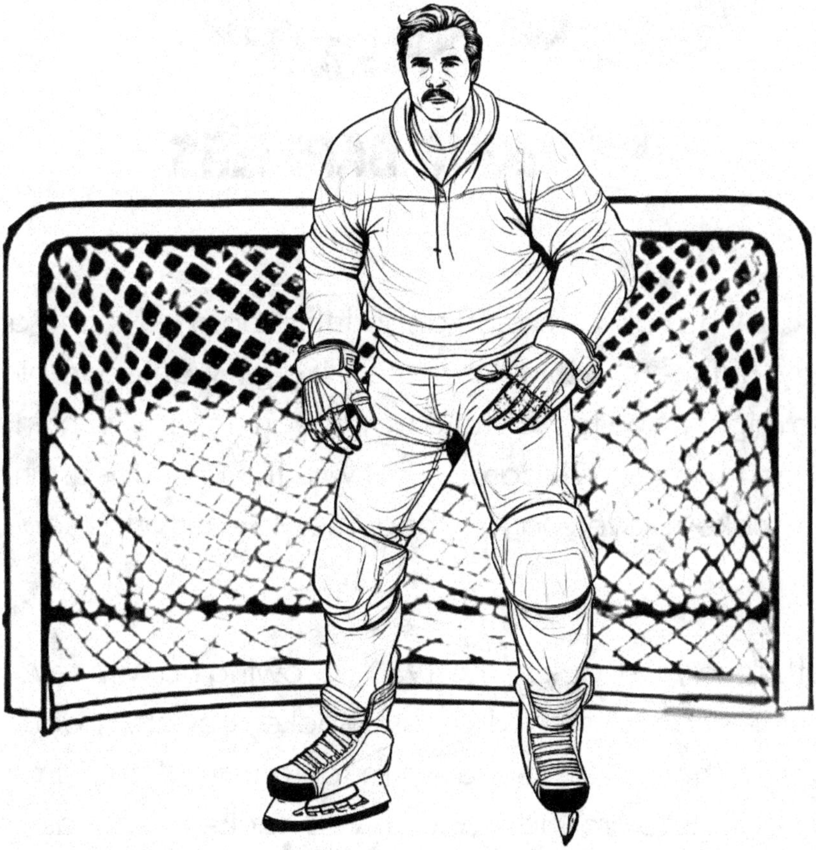

CHAPTER 8

BREAKING BARRIERS

Hockey has always been a sport that both boys and girls play. But there was a time when, if a girl wanted to play, she might have to look for a boy's team to play with since all-girl teams were scarce. That was the case for aspiring ice hockey player Manon Rheaume of Beauport, Quebec.

Let's take you back to the 1980s. Growing up with several brothers and a father who was a hockey coach, Rheaume took to the sport that was so much a part of her family's life. Everyone around Manon loved hockey, so it was only natural that she fell in love with the sport. Whenever a team needed a goalie for a local tournament, her father agreed to let her play, and it quickly became evident that she was good. Rheaume had a real gift for hockey, and she was over the moon that she was finally getting the recognition she deserved. Like we said, female hockey players were few and far between at the time.

As she got older, many teams sought out her goaltending services. When she was 11 years old (yes! She was only 11 at this point!), she got a chance to play in the Quebec City International Pee Wee Tournament, an event that has seen many of its participants go on to careers in the National Hockey League. She was the first girl ever to play in the prestigious tournament—Rheaume's making history.

In 1991, when she turned 19, Rheaume was an outstanding goalie, so good in fact that she got an opportunity to play with the Trois-Rivières Draveurs of the Quebec Major Junior Hockey League, one of the top junior hockey leagues in the world and one that has produced talents such as Guy Lafleur, Mario Lemieux, and Sydney Crosby.

She got her chance to play when she was sent in the second period of a tied game. The first shot she faced hit her in the mask, causing her head to bleed. Undaunted, she stayed in the game. While she only played three games for Les Draveurs, it put her name on the map, and it wasn't long before professional teams wanted her to play for them. One of those teams was the NHL's newest team, the Tampa Bay Lightning.

While the move was part of a publicity stunt to get some local interest in the new team, management insisted that Rheaume was there because of her talent. That fall, during the exhibition season, Rheaume played one period of a game against the St. Louis Blues. Although she gave up two goals on nine shots, she became the first woman to play a game in any of the four major sports leagues in North America.

She would bounce around various men's leagues but never managed to stick around very long, although she did earn her first professional win with the Knoxville Cherokees of the East Coast Hockey League. By this point, women's hockey had grown in stature, and with her professional experience, she was a natural to join Team Canada. As a national team member, she won two World Championships and a silver medal at the 1996 Olympics.

Today, she works for the Los Angeles Kings. But it all started because a boy's team needed a goalie.

Manon Rheaume's legacy is something to be inspired by, particularly for young girls with big dreams. Surrounded by brothers who loved hockey, she may have felt like an underdog as the only girl. But let this be an important lesson in empowerment. Despite all the odds and setbacks she faced, Manon went on to become a legend in not only women's hockey but hockey as a whole.

Do you have dreams that you feel like you're being held back from? Let it be known that you are as capable as boys to achieve anything you want. Whether you dream of becoming a professional athlete or running your own business, this world is yours for the taking.

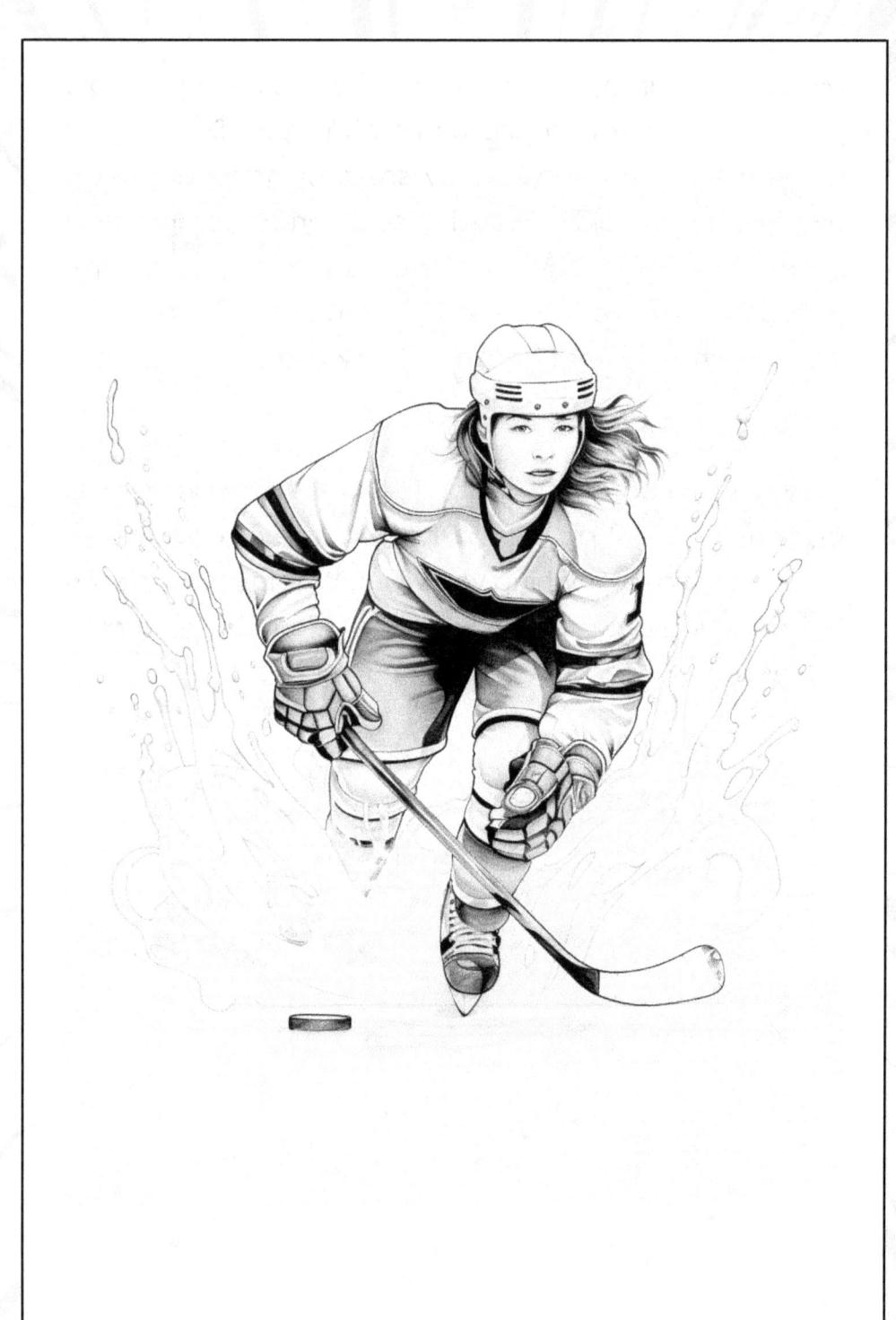

CHAPTER 9

TALES OF THE STANLEY CUP

When the final buzzer sounds or the winning goal hits the back of the net, the celebration that follows a Stanley Cup win sends both players into a frenzy. When the Cup is presented, the players skate around the ice, have a team photo taken, and then the party begins.

But what happens after the locker room celebrations and parades are over? Well, every player on the winning team gets their day with the Cup; a day when they can choose to take the trophy wherever they want and share it with family, friends, and fans. If only that Cup could talk.

When it was first presented in 1893, few knew what kind of ride the silver rose bowl Lord Stanley of Preston bought for ten guineas or about $50 would go on. The first winners, the Montreal Amateur Athletic Association, added the first ring to the bottom of the bowl to add their team's name. As more teams won, more names were added to the ring. When space became tight, names were engraved on the bowl itself, first outside, then inside the bowl.

Over the years, more rings were added, and the names of the players and coaches were included. The Cup soon became very tall and thin and was referred to as the stovepipe or elephant's leg Cup. After the 1947 season, it was redesigned to look like today's trophy. In 1956, with the original Cup becoming brittle and the rings full, a new, redesigned Cup was created. New, wider bands designed for 13 championship teams' names and players' names were created. When a ring is full, a new ring is added, and the top ring is removed and placed in the Hockey Hall of Fame.

To get your name included with a winning team, you must have played at least 41 games with the team in the regular season and be with the team when they win or at least one game in the Stanley Cup Finals. Up to 52 names can be added, including coaches and support staff.

Over the years, the Cup has taken quite a beating as jubilant players made some poor decisions with the trophy. In 1905, Ottawa Senators players tried to kick the Cup across the Rideau Canal. It ended up stuck in the ice. In 1926, on their way to a party, players from the Montreal Canadiens stopped to fix a flat tire in the car they were driving in. They left the Cup on the sidewalk and drove away. Once they realized their mistake, they rushed back to find the Cup right where they left it.

In the years since, it has been in swimming pools and nightclubs, traveled overseas, and the New York Rangers' burned their mortgage in the bowl.

And who, you might ask, has his name on the Cup the most? Jean Beliveau has been there 18 times, 10 as a player with the Montreal Canadiens and 8 as an executive with the team.

The great thing about the Stanley Cup, as we've learned, is that it's pretty much been everywhere—most teams have had it at some point. So, what can we take from this?

Just because you lose doesn't mean you won't win one day. And vice versa—don't be too prideful in winning all the time because the trophy may be passed on one day. It's important to accept that both losing and winning are great things. And, hey, who knows? Maybe one day, the Stanley Cup will be yours.

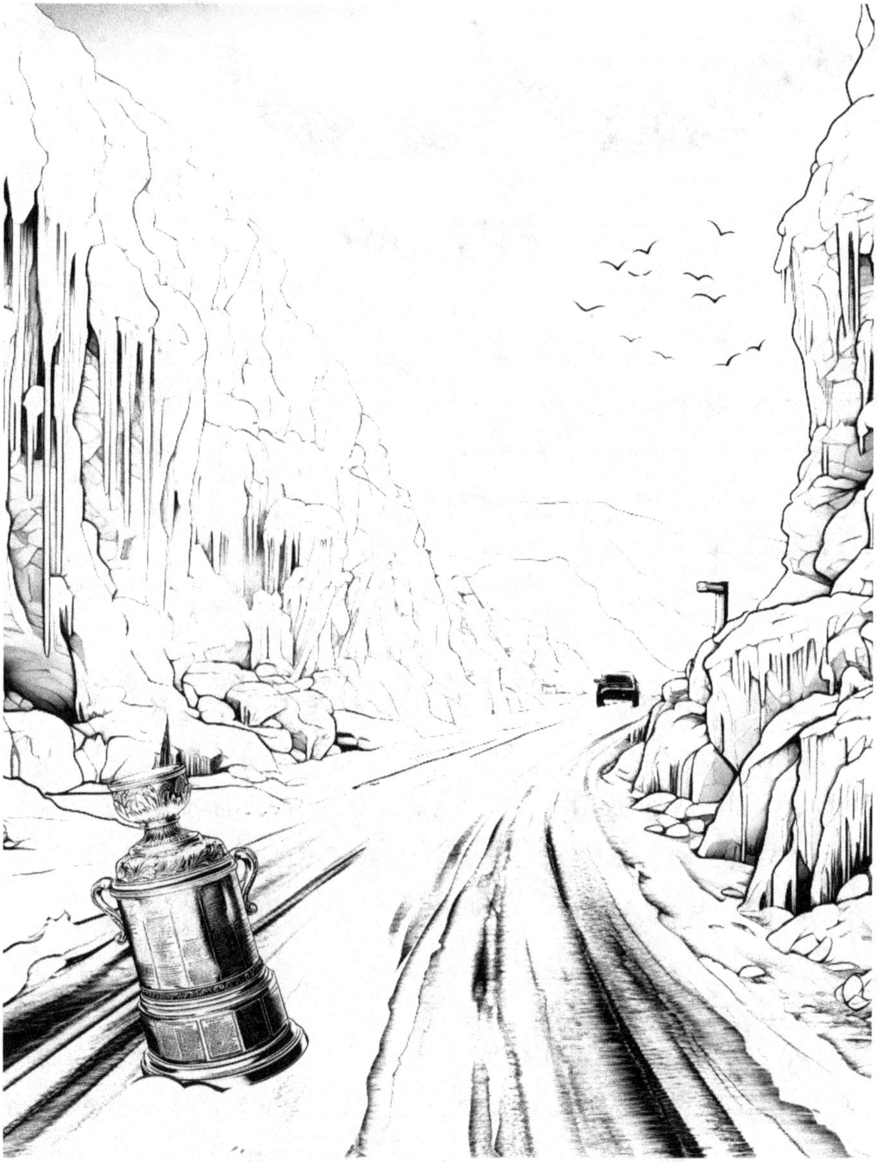

CHAPTER 10

BATMAN

It is not often that someone or something distracts thousands of fans in the arena from what is happening on the ice. During the 1975 Stanley Cup finals, a bat would almost steal the show. Yes, a bat!

That spring, the Philadelphia Flyers were trying to win their second straight Stanley Cup and faced the upstart Buffalo Sabres in the finals. The Sabres were only in their fifth season in the league, while the Flyers had become the first non-original six team to win the title.

The Flyers' home arena was the Philadelphia Spectrum, one of the NHL's most modern buildings and one built specifically for the team. It was state of the art at the time and had a key feature of air conditioning. On the other hand, the Sabers played in the Buffalo Auditorium, built in 1940 and lacked modern amenities.

When game three and the series moved to Buffalo, the temperatures outside soared to 28C or 82F, warm for May in northern New York state. With over 16,000 fans in attendance inside the arena, the temperatures continued to rise, as did the humidity. The game started as usual, but a layer of fog soon developed over the ice. Not long afterward, the lower half of the player's legs began disappearing into the mist, and it became tough for fans on TV and in person to follow the game. Fans in the arena were squinting, hoping the fog would clear so they wouldn't miss any of the game.

The game started to take on an eerie look and feel, looking more like Halloween than mid-spring. Then, almost on cue, a bat flew down from the rafters and started circling the ice. Many figured the bat was trying to escape the heat building up in the roof of the old arena. As the game went on, the bat buzzed the players. Then the bat decided to get a closer look at the players, coming in while they were lining up for a face-off. That's when Buffalo's Jim Lorentz took matters into his own hands and whacked the bat out of the air with his stick. From that moment on, Lorentz had a new nickname with the Sabres: Batman.

Even though the bat caused trouble for the players on the rink, it was absolutely hilarious to the audience. Feeling a little disappointed by the poor vision, they finally had something to keep them entertained. This little moment of pure coincidence, where nature collided with sport, changed an eerie and blurred vision into a memorable moment in hockey history.

What has this tiny bat taught us? Even if things in life are looking foggy (metaphorically, that is), a little glimmer of hope or a slight touch of humor always finds its way through the fog to lighten the mood a little.

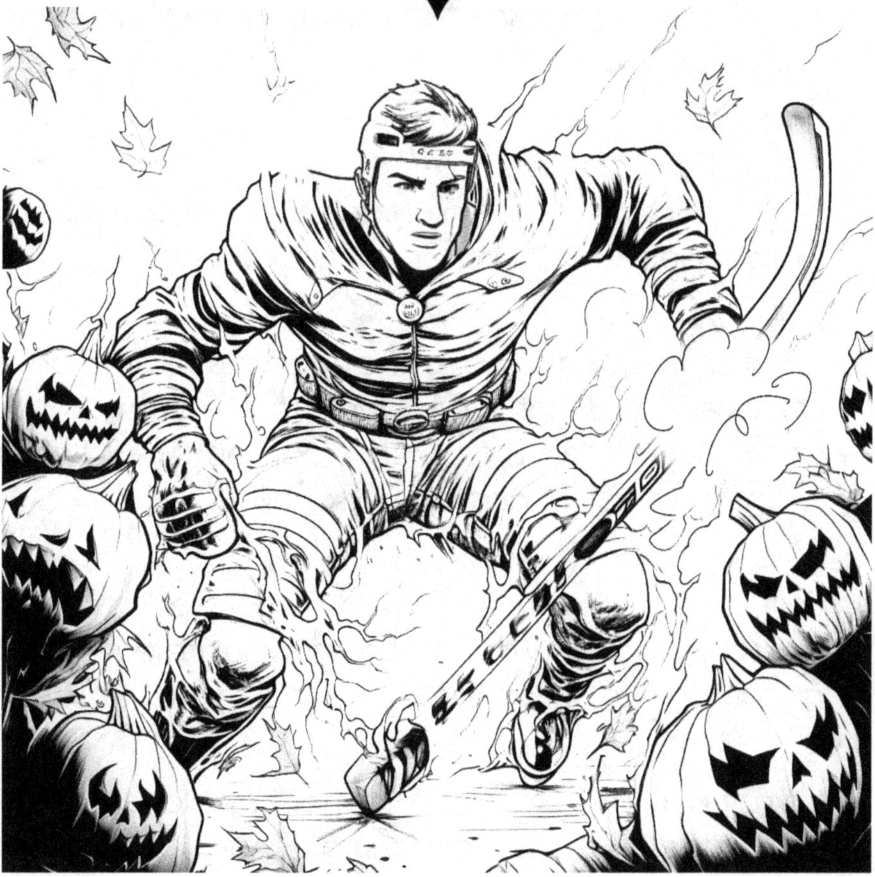

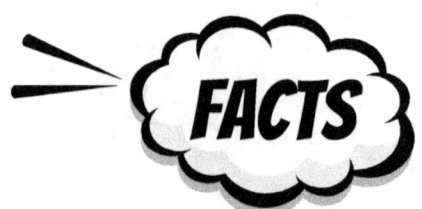

1. Early hockey players did not wear helmets, and the NHL did not make helmets required for new players until 1979. Goalkeepers used to play without face masks!

2. A guest is frequently invited to drop the puck for the ceremonial faceoff before each game. It could be a famous person, a local hero, or a fan.

3. Goalies frequently have the most distinctive and creative mask designs. The artwork, ranging from movie characters to team emblems, can be as wild and imaginative as the goalie's personality.

4. Early hockey sticks were made of wood, but modern sticks are commonly made of composite materials such as carbon fiber for enhanced durability and flexibility.

5. It's not only a stereotype that hockey players have missing teeth. Because of the intensity and fast-paced nature of the game, players occasionally lose a tooth or two on the ice.

CHAPTER 11

MEETING YOUR IDOL

When you start playing hockey, it is natural to want to imitate your on-ice heroes. I mean, they all say you should learn from the best, right? Whether it is their style of play, how they skate, or even how they might tape their stick or lace their skates, copying your idols is as old as the game itself. And sometimes, your heroes take notice.

Growing up in Thurso, Quebec, Guy Lafleur's skill and ability was already getting him noticed when he was a kid. Some were even labeling him as a player who was destined to make the NHL. Like most kids in Quebec, he was a fan of the Montreal Canadiens, and his idol was the Habs' captain, Jean Beliveau. Young Guy would try to play like the big, smooth-skating center and even wore his famous number four. Think about it: a lot of people do similar things, too. Maybe you wear your favorite singer's merch, or perhaps you're learning to draw the way your favorite artist does. But none of us think we'll ever get the chance to meet our idol, do we?

When Guy was just 12 years old, he played in the famous Quebec City Pee Wee Hockey Tournament. It was the same tournament Manon Rheaume played in at 11 years old. Games would be played at the Quebec Coliseum, the arena built to accommodate fans who wanted to watch Guy's idol Beliveau when he played in Quebec as an amateur. So, there Guy is, playing in the very same stadium that his idol used to play at all the time. And who was there watching from the sides? You guessed it, Jean Beliveau himself.

When Lafleur scored a hat trick in a game, Beliveau presented Guy with the Player of the Game award. What a thrill for Lafleur! He had finally met his idol. Someone he had admired for years recognized Guy's skills and awarded him for it. As Beliveau met the star-struck youngster, he told him that one day, he might play for the Canadiens. Guy was delighted to hear this and continued to work hard to achieve that goal one day. Eight years later, that would come true as Lafleur was drafted by Montreal. When his career was over, Lafleur had scored more points than any other player in Montreal history, beating the record set by, you guessed it, Jean Beliveau.

Guy Lafleur, who had previously only ever dreamed of becoming even half as good as Jean Beliveau, became a renowned ice hockey star and, of course, an inspiration to many kids to come.

Lafleur teaches us that it is so important to never give up on your dreams. What's a big ambition you have? What would you really love to do when you get older? Do you have an idol that you look up to? Well, take a page out of Lafleur's book and keep on pushing to achieve that dream. And, hey, you never know; you may just meet your idol.

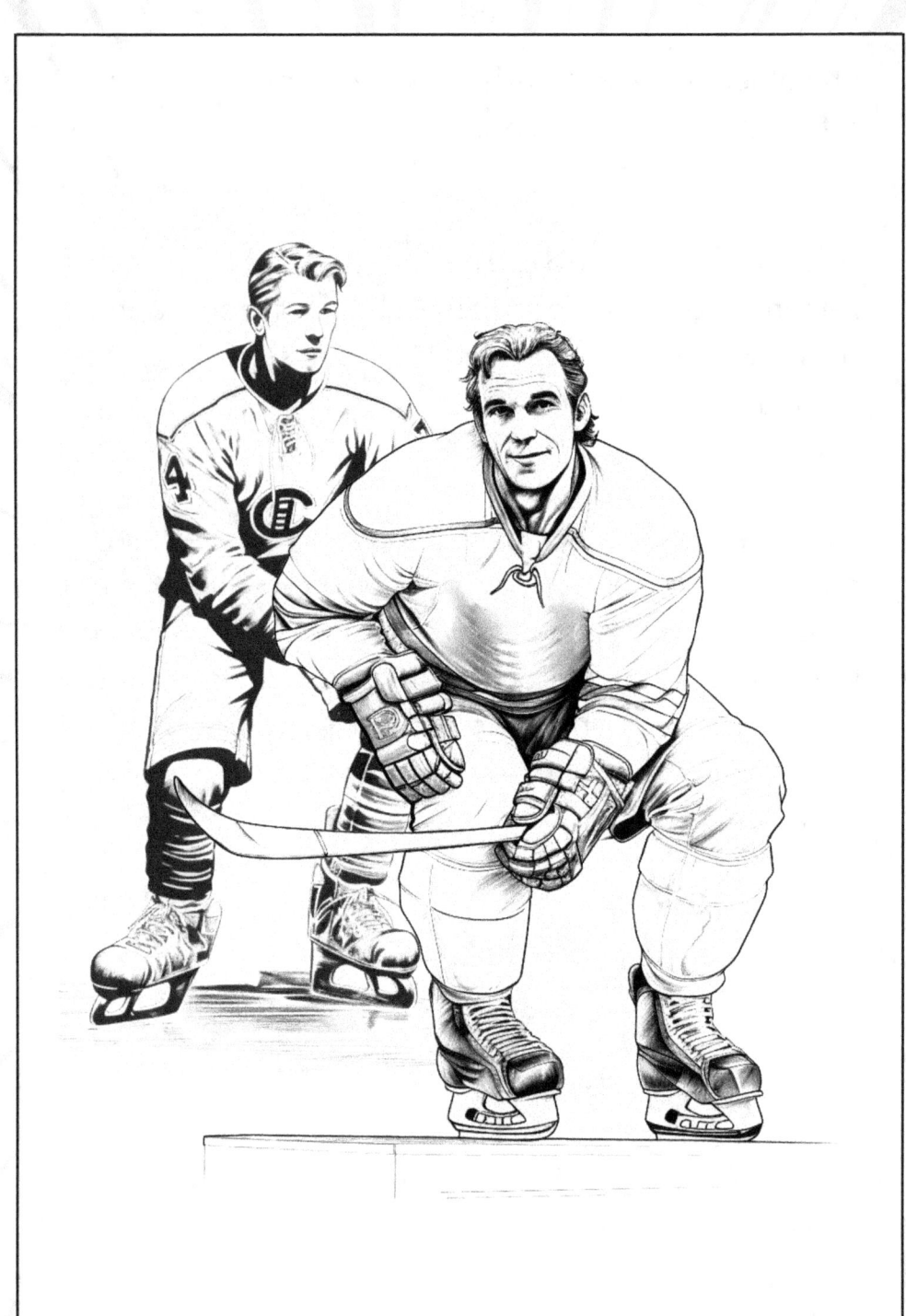

CHAPTER 12

THE ROCKET NETS FIVE - TWICE!

Have you ever been asked to do something you didn't want to do? That was the case in December of 1944 when Maurice 'The Rocket' Richard was called into action for a game he wasn't even supposed to play.

The game was against the Detroit Red Wings in the middle of a cold Montreal winter. The day before, Richard had spent time moving him and his wife from one apartment to another. The move, up and down Montreal's famous tall staircases, had taken its toll on Richard, and he was exhausted. His coach, Dick Irvin Sr., had promised him he could miss the Detroit game to rest up from the move. But as game time approached, the phone in Richard's new home rang, and the coach told him he needed to play.

With Montreal and Detroit having almost identical records, Irving knew the game was important, even if it was still early in the season. Dutifully, a tired Richard arrived at the Montreal Forum and put on his famous number '9' jersey.

By the end of the first period, Richard had a goal and an assist, already a decent night's work for any player. In the second period, Richard would score two goals in eight seconds for the hat trick, then add another goal and an assist. In just 40 minutes, The Rocket was sitting on a six-point night. In the third, he would add one more goal and another assist for a five-goal, eight-point night as the Canadiens thumped the Red Wings 9-1. The eight points in one game remains a Montreal record.

Later that spring, as the Canadiens faced their bitter rivals, the Toronto Maple Leafs, in the playoffs, it would once again be Richard's time to shine. After a game-one victory by the Leafs, the Canadiens were desperate for a win. Not wanting to fall further behind, Richard put the Habs on his back and, with help from his linemates Elmer Lach and Hector 'Toe' Blake, Richard would once again net five goals for a 5-1 Montreal win.

When it came time to announce the game's three stars, the Montreal fans were shocked when the third star was announced as Maurice Richard. After a performance they'd witnessed, this was a slap in the face. Then the second star was announced: Maurice Richard. And the first star? Maurice Richard. One of the local newspapers even ran the headline Richard 5, Maple Leafs 1.

It was the first time in modern NHL history that five goals were scored in a playoff game and the first time a player was named all three stars.

We've all been there, right? Someone has asked us to do something that we don't feel like doing. Maybe we can't be bothered or don't feel like helping, but let's learn something from The Rocket.

His team really needed him that night, and he came through for them despite not feeling his best—and who knows if they could've won without him? So, next time you're asked to help a friend, family member, or team out, be like The Rocket.

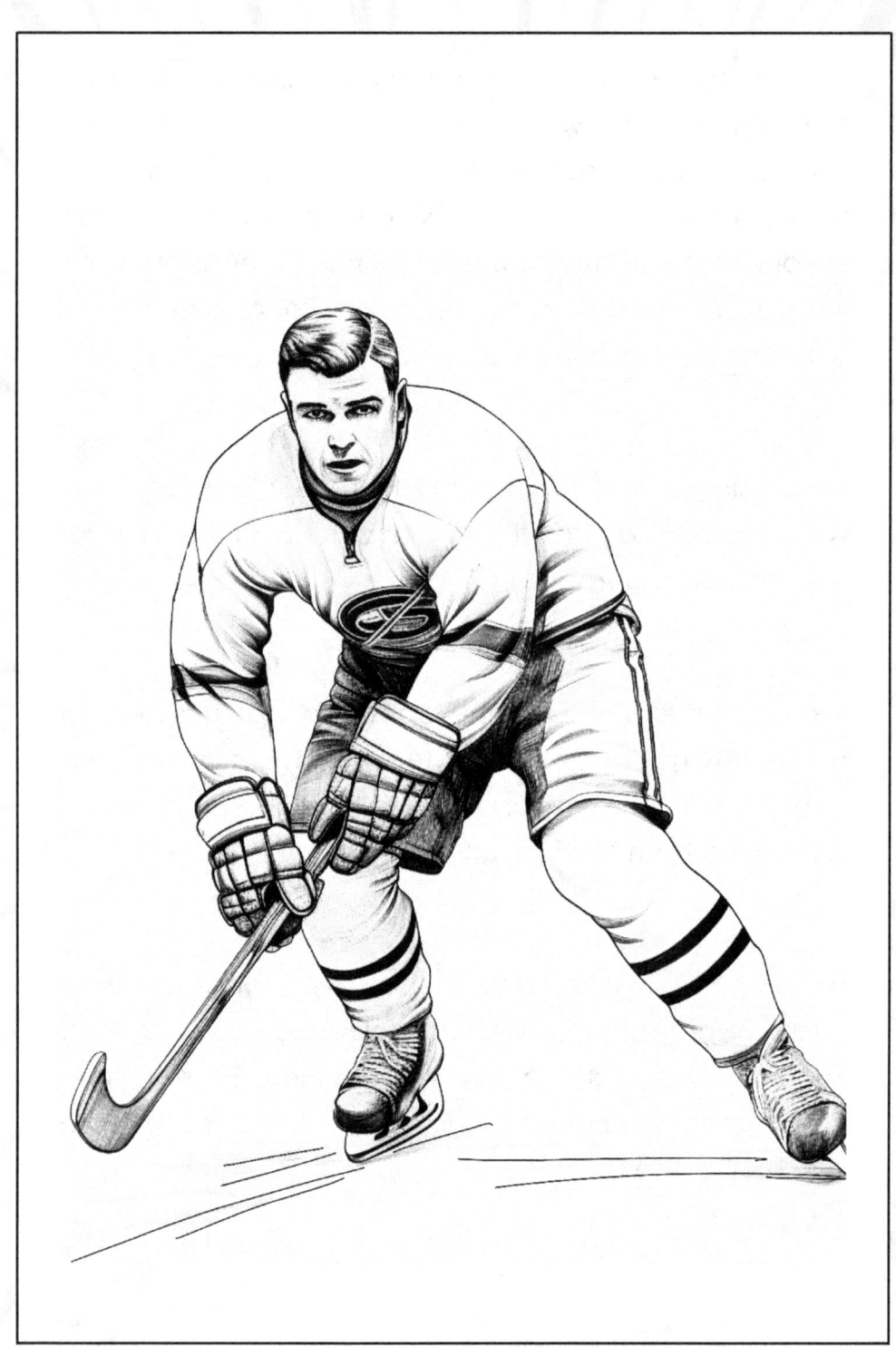

CHAPTER 13

GEARED UP

No sport in the world requires more equipment than hockey. Whether you are playing as a forward or defenceman, you have a complete set of protection you must put on before skating out onto the ice. You will need even more if you are a goalie. But how did this come about?

The evolution of hockey equipment is as old as the game itself. While the origins of the game are lost in time (some say it was invented in Montreal, others in Nova Scotia), the one basic piece of equipment was skates. But these weren't the skates you are used to today; they were a blade that strapped onto your boots or shoes. Sticks were whatever you could find, usually a stick or a cane.

Padding didn't emerge for several years, and the first area people protected was their shins. Players would put pieces of wood in their socks or, more commonly, old magazines or newspapers because they could wrap around their legs.

And when it came to pucks, anything that slid on the ice was good enough. Once again, blocks of wood were common, as were something called a horse apple. These were horse droppings that could be found on any road since horses were still widely in use for delivering items like milk, coal, and ice. When a horse pooped in winter, their poop would freeze, making for a perfect substitute puck.

Helmets were not common, although a few players wore them after getting a head injury. But the rule requiring all players to wear a helmet didn't start until 1979. It wasn't until 2013 that all players entering the NHL had to wear a visor.

Goalies had to make do with whatever they could find to help protect them. What we consider goalie pads today originated from the English game of cricket. There, players who are at bat wear leg pads to protect them from the ball, and they are perfect for hockey. Masks, on the other hand, were different.

While they'd been experimented with in the 1920s and '30s, most goalies never wore masks, including Montreal Canadiens goalie Jacques Plante. Even though he'd played many all-star seasons without a mask, it always made him feel uncomfortable. He began experimenting with a fiberglass mask in practice, but his coach, Toe Blake, refused to let him wear it in games.

That changed on November 1, 1959, when, in a game against the New York Rangers, Plante was hit in the face with a shot from Rangers star Andy Bathgate. Cut across his nose, Plante was stitched up but refused to return to the ice without the mask. Having no alternative, his coach let him wear the mask, and hockey was forever changed. Many goalies adopted the mask, but a few held out. The last goalie to not wear a mask in a game was Andy Brown of the Pittsburgh Penguins. Today, if a goalie's mask is knocked off, play stops immediately.

These mishaps, especially Plante's, teach us about the importance of safety. It shows us why certain rules are put in place—to keep you safe! That's why we wear bike helmets, buckle our seatbelts in the car, or wear kneepads when rollerblading. Without safety procedures, we are vulnerable to injuries.

Safety first!

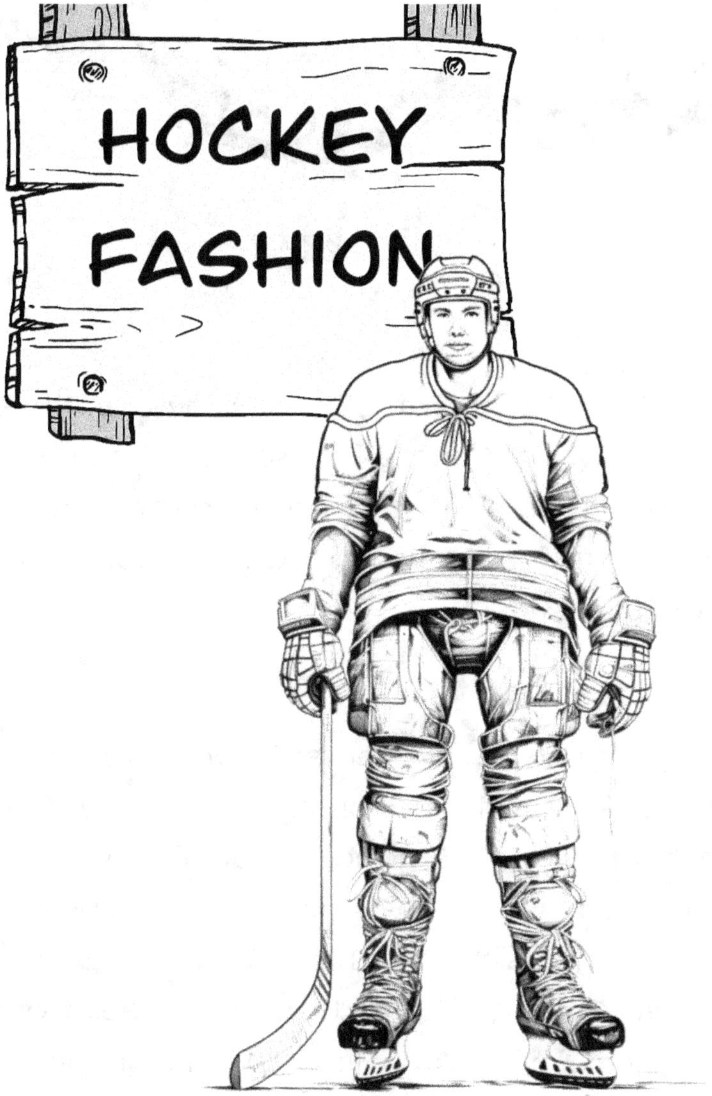

HOCKEY FASHION

CHAPTER 14

UPSET

When the 2006 Winter Olympics rolled around, the eyes of the hockey world were focused on the Women's Tournament. Making only its third appearance at the Games, the previous two finals featured Team Canada and Team USA.

In 1998, in the first-ever Women's Olympic Final, the Americans stunned the favored Canadians 7-4 in the gold medal game at Nagano, Japan. Four years later, in Salt Lake City, Utah, it was the Americans who were picked to win gold since they had the home advantage. Despite some questionable calls by the referees, Canada held on for a 3-2 win. Now, with the Games in Turin, Italy, the teams were set for another battle between the North American neighbors.

Everyone except the team from Sweden.

The tournament began as expected. Canada pounded the host Italians 16-0, then trounced Russia 12-0, followed by the Swedes 8-1. On the other side of the bracket, Team USA beat Switzerland 6-0, Germany 5-0, and Finland 7-3. Since the Americans and Canadians finished atop their respective groups, they would face the second-place team from the other division in the semifinals.

Canada made short work of the plucky Finns, blanking them 6-0 to advance to the gold medal game. As far as everyone was concerned, the Americans would do the same, and the rubber match of gold medal games would take place.

When the game started, the Americans blitzed the Swedish net, but goalie Kim Martin stood her ground as best she could, allowing only one power-play goal in the first period for a somewhat surprising 1-0 USA lead.

The Americans doubled their lead early in the second, but a goal from Sweden's Maria Rooth five minutes later gave the Swedes hope. That hope turned to belief when Rooth scored her second of the game three minutes later.

After a scoreless third, the game went into overtime, and again, no goals were scored. That meant a shootout. The Swedes, now brimming with confidence, put all their hope in their shooters and Martin, who had stopped 37 shots in the game.

After the first two Swedish and American shooters failed to score, Pernilla Winberg scored to give the Swedes a 1-0 lead. The next shooter was American captain Krissy Wendel, who was stopped by Martin. The next Swedish shooter was Martin. If she scored, the game was over. And she did. The Swedes had upset the balance of Women's hockey.

Canada would win the gold, beating Sweden 4-1, but the silver medal might as well have been gold for the Swedes. They had shown the world that Women's Hockey was more than Canada and the USA and proved that they belonged as well.

You may, like the Swedes, feel underestimated by people who have more recognition or are seemingly better than you at something. Just like them, you should keep pushing to prove yourself despite odds and setbacks. You deserve to be recognized for your worth—so fight for it!

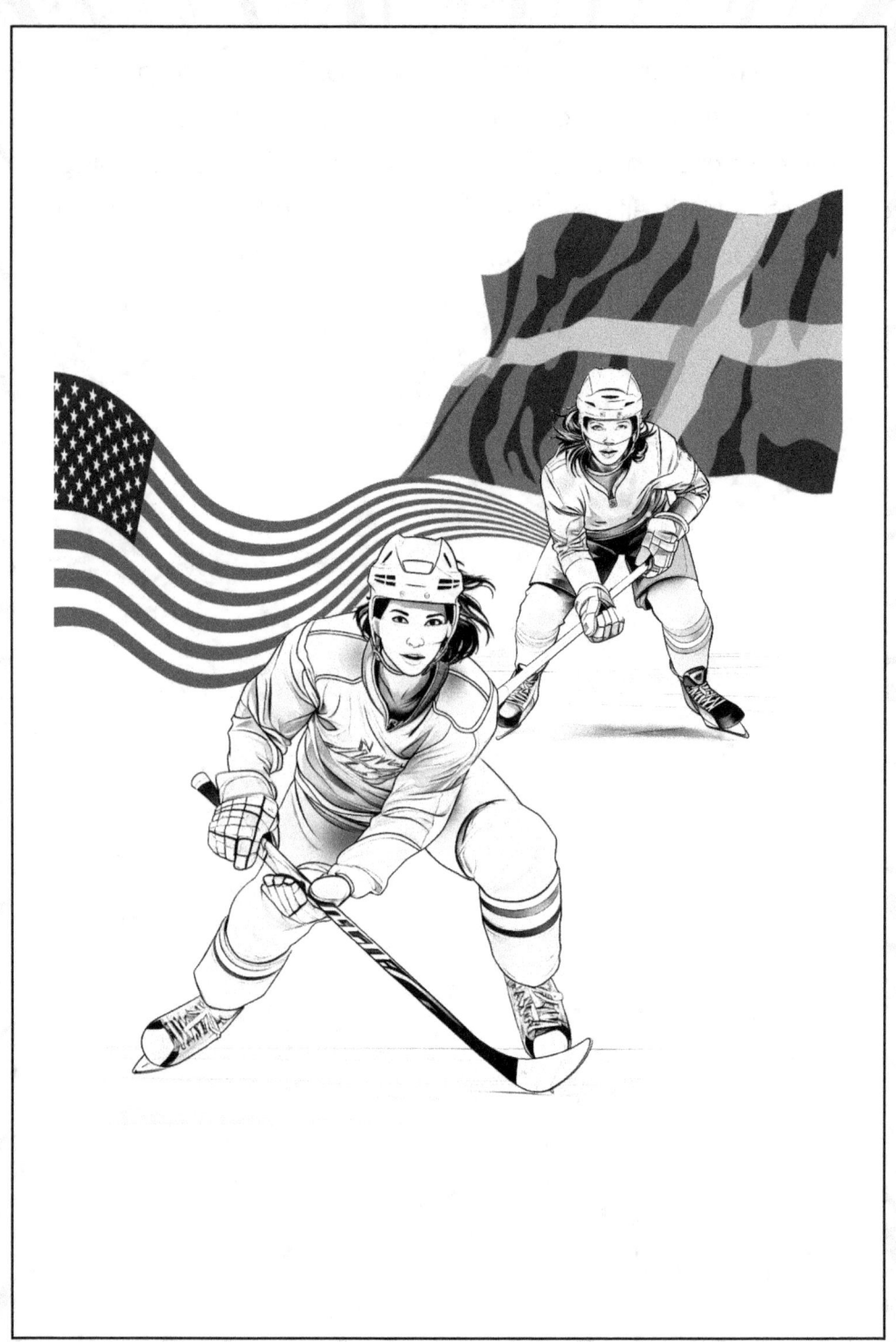

CHAPTER 15

TOOTOO

It is a long way from the Canadian Territory of Nunavut, located near the Arctic Circle, to basically anywhere. For Jordin Tootoo, making the trip from Rankin Inlet to the NHL was a long but worthwhile journey.

For Tootoo, this journey began when he was just 13 years old when he made the 1,700 km journey from Rankin Inlet to Spruce Grove, Alberta—he wasn't going to let distance get in the way. Wanting to play high-level hockey, Spruce Grove was a good option for the young player. It's said that Tootoo was bullied by his peers at this time for being an Inuit and often felt like an outsider—how awful is that? As an Inuit, he was able to billet with a First Nations family, making the transition easier. In his new home, Jordin played Bantam AAA, the highest level of hockey for that age group.

While it was tough to make the adjustment, young Jordin thrived with his new team and eventually caught the eye of junior hockey scouts from the Western Hockey League, one of Canada's three Major Junior hockey leagues. He was good enough that the Brandon Wheat Kings, one of Canada's oldest and most storied junior teams, were keen to get him on their team. In 2003, at 20 years old, he was chosen to represent Canada at the World Junior Hockey Championships, helping Canada win a silver medal.

After a year of seasoning with the ONC Blizzard in the Manitoba Junior 'A' league, Jordin started a four-year career with Brandon. Playing in the WHL can be tough. Long bus rides from the middle of Canada to the West Coast of both Canada and the United States and having to balance hockey and school didn't faze Jordin, and he would soon become a team leader. Known for his scrappy style and ability to get under opposing players' skin, he was also a contributor on offense and a team leader. Those qualities and a 'never give up' attitude attracted notice from the NHL.

At the 2001 NHL Draft, Jordin was selected with the first pick of the fourth round by the Nashville Predators. It would be a year and a half before he made his NHL debut, but the wait was worth it. On October 9, 2003 – wearing number 22, like his name – Jordin skated onto the ice to face the Mighty Ducks of Anaheim. He became the first person of Inuit descent to play in the NHL, making incredible history for his indigenous community. Imagine how proud everyone was!

It didn't take long for Jordin to become a fan favorite, as Nashville fans fell in love with his hard-nosed style. He also became an advocate for cultural integrity and spoke to youth about the importance of upholding your community. One week after his debut, he scored his first career goal against the Atlanta Thrashers.

Over the next 13 seasons, Tootoo became one of the most popular players in the NHL, especially within the First Nations community. After Nashville, he would play with New Jersey, Detroit, and Chicago. Since retiring from the NHL, he has helped grow the sport of hockey throughout the Inuit community while raising money to help kids who are dealing with personal issues.

For a kid from the edge of the world, he has certainly left his mark on the sport. The NHL celebrated Tootoo's indigenous culture, and his various teams would learn a lot from his strength and determination. This goes to show that, despite odds and circumstances, we can achieve great things and that our individual cultures should be celebrated.

Tootoo's story also teaches us a valuable lesson that we should never bully others for being 'different'. We all come from different backgrounds, have our own strengths and weaknesses, and bring new things to the table. Even if someone seems a little different, you should treat them with the same respect.

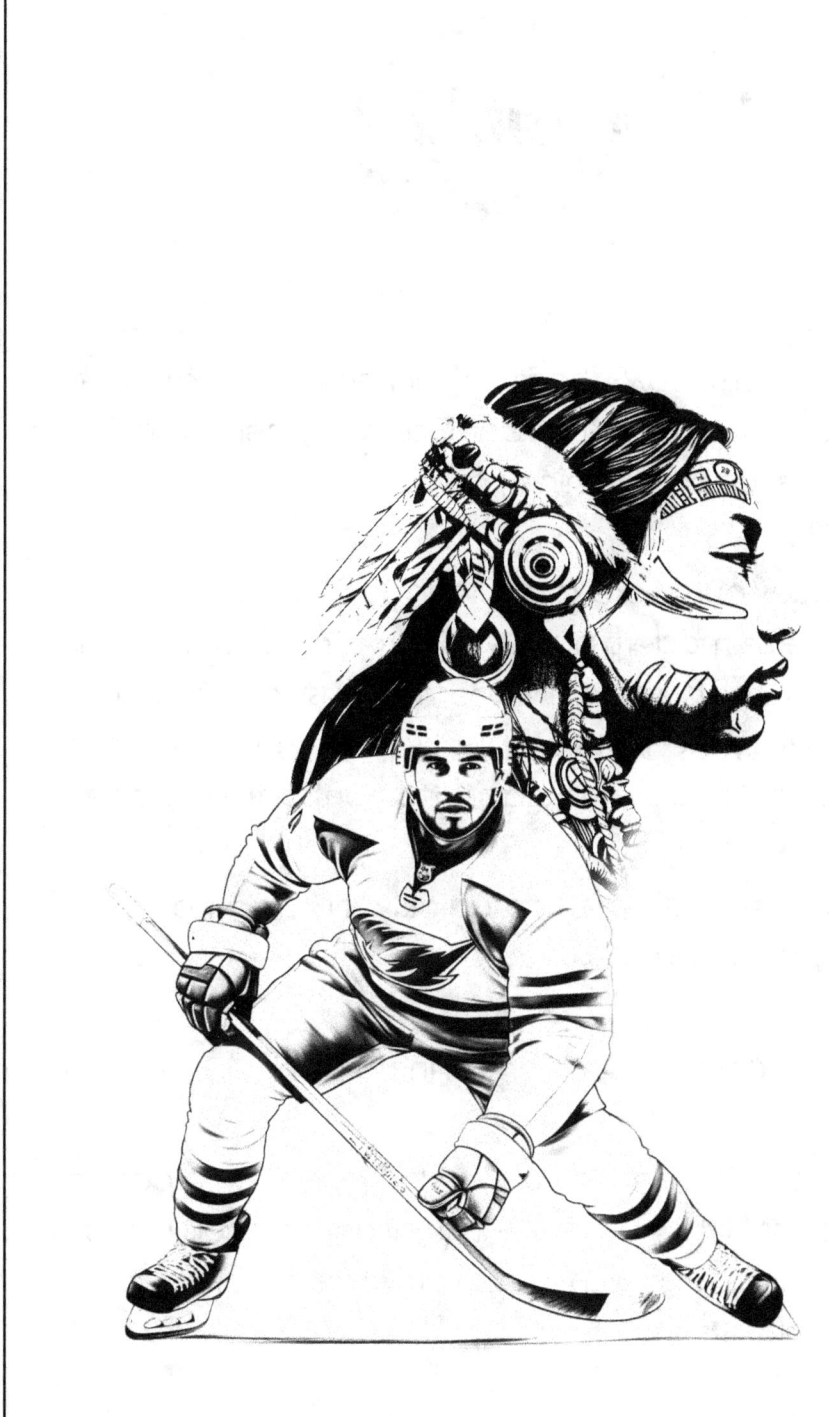

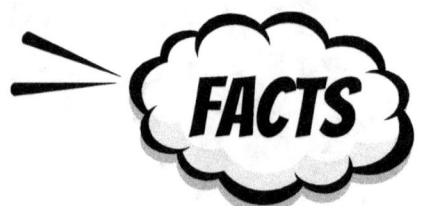

FACTS

1. On March 3, 1875, the first organized indoor ice hockey game began in Montreal, Canada. There were two teams, each with nine players.

2. Hockey pucks are kept frozen until they are used in a game. A modern puck is constructed of rubber, and when it gets warm, it becomes flimsy and bounces. Freezing the hockey pucks prevents them from bouncing, allowing players to control them better.

3. Because they melt so quickly, NHL games often employ 12 pucks.

4. The rink's ice is less than an inch thick.

5. Some teams employ players known as "enforcers" or "goons" who specialize in fighting and violent play. Their job is to guard top players while also intimidating opponents.

CHAPTER 16

NUMBER FOUR, BOBBY ORR

Occasionally, a player who is deemed a 'generational' player comes along. This usually means he is a lock to not only make the NHL but have an impact on the game. The most recent example would be Edmonton's Connor McDavid. In the early 1960s, that player was a tall kid from Parry Sound, Ontario, named Bobby Orr.

Orr was a youth hockey player before the days of the NHL draft, which meant any team could sign him if he, or better yet, his family, agreed. As Montreal, Detroit, and Toronto made offers, the Boston Bruins would sign the young Orr. The Bruins gave Orr's minor team $1,000 (about $10,000 today) and planned to start a new junior team in Oshawa, Ontario, with Orr as the centerpiece. The team would be named the Generals in honor of Oshawa's top employer and sponsor, General Motors. The one concern was Orr was still only 14, and most junior players were between 18 and 20.

There was also the issue of leaving home. Orr's mother didn't want her young son so far away, so an arrangement was made to have him make the three-hour drive south for games. Despite only playing 34 games and being the target of older and bigger players who resented the attention Orr was getting, he managed six goals and 21 points.

A year later, having grown and with a year's experience, Orr started to show the style that would allow him to change the game. At that time, defencemen weren't known for their offense, but the slick-skating Orr changed that, setting a junior hockey record with 29 goals and 43 assists. He would break his own record each of the next two seasons.

At 18, the Bruins decided it was time to cash in on their investment, and Orr was called up to the NHL. After wearing number 2 in junior, Orr switched to 4 since 2 had been retired by the Bruins. At the time, the Bruins were at the bottom of the six-team NHL, but they had Orr and many more young, talented players on the way. With a 41-point season, Orr won the Calder Trophy as the league's top rookie and was considered for the Norris Trophy for top defenceman. Winner Harry Howell said he was glad to win it because Orr would soon own the trophy. He won it for the next eight years straight.

Like in junior, Orr revolutionized how defense was played. Before Orr, defencemen rarely got more than 40 points in a season and were recognized for not allowing goals more than scoring them. In only his fourth year, he would register 120 points, leading Boston to their first Stanley Cup in 29 years, scoring the cup-winning goal in overtime. The next season, he'd set another record with 102 assists, the first player ever to record more than 100 in a season.

By 1975, injuries had taken a toll on Orr. At only 28, he moved to the Chicago Blackhawks but would play only 26 games for them over two seasons. In one final hurrah, Orr played for Canada at the 1976 Canada Cup. On a team and tournament full of stars, Orr was named MVP as Canada won the championship. Despite knee injuries that made it painful to walk, Canada teammate Daryl Sittler said, "Bobby was better on one leg than most players are on two".

Orr's story goes to show that you can still achieve great things despite your age. He was always the youngest player wherever he went. Many underestimated his abilities, thinking he was a laughing stock because he was so young, but, oh boy, did Orr prove them wrong.

You may hear people say that you're too young to be dreaming big, but let Orr be a great example that just because you're young doesn't mean you can't start chasing your dreams.

4

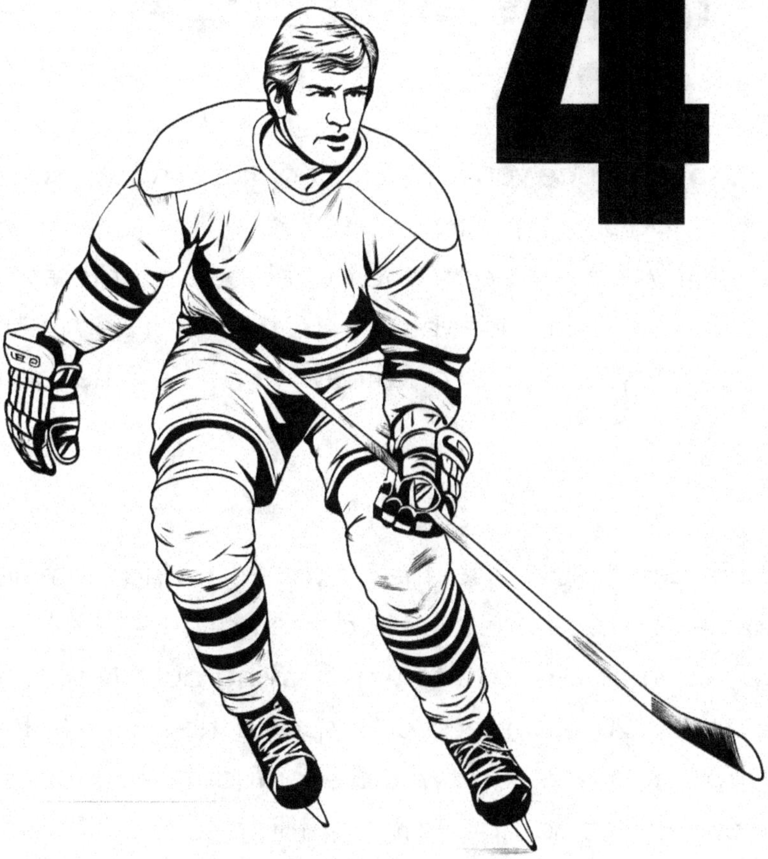

CHAPTER 17

IT'S OKAY NOT TO BE OKAY

Allow us to introduce you to NHL ice hockey forward player for the Tampa Bay Lightnings, Tyler Motte. Motte grew up in a small town in Michigan and developed an interest in hockey because his older brother, C.J., was a goalie–he was inspired by his brother and knew he wanted the same career for himself.

He soon started playing for the Detroit Red Wings, a minor ice hockey team, in the Quebec International Pee-Wee Hockey Tournament. Motte was moving quickly up the ranks, and, in 2016, he secured a spot in the NHL with the Chicago Blackhawks and would eventually permanently end up with the Tampa Bay Lightning team. Life was seemingly perfect for Motte–he finally had everything he dreamed of. But things are never as they seem, and, as it turns out, Motte had been silently suffering with something for a long time.

In 2020, Motte shared that he had recently been diagnosed with anxiety and depression. His doctors said in a routine check-up that, physically, he was in perfect shape. All his limbs worked perfectly fine, he had no underlying health conditions, and everything seemed to be a-okay for this star ice hockey player. But when the doctors asked if there was anything else they could help with, Motte opened up about his mental health struggles.

Since his diagnosis, Motte has been a huge advocate for openly discussing mental health and is constantly sharing heartfelt and honest conversations all over social media. People talk a lot about physical health, but mental health has always been a little different. Often, we shy away from sharing if we're struggling mentally—maybe we've been conditioned to keep these things to ourselves; who knows?

But let Motte's story be a lesson that it's okay, and completely normal, to open up about how you're feeling. It's okay to ask for help, and it's important to remember that you have a lot of people in your life who are willing and ready to listen.

Don't suffer in silence and carry this alone. Trust me, as soon as you open up, you'll feel a huge weight lifted off your shoulders. Mental health is so important, so we hope Motte's story helps you feel able to talk about it openly.

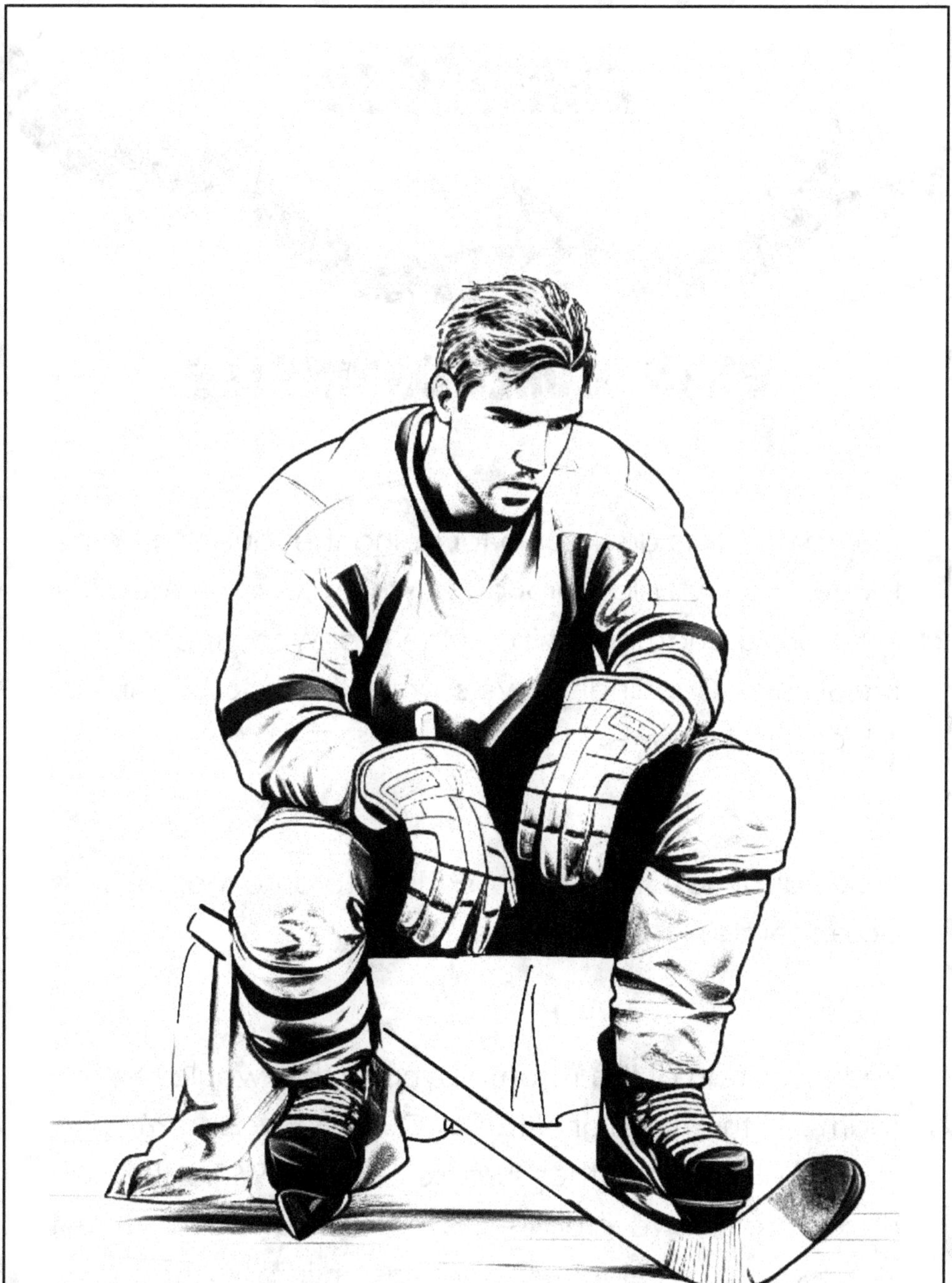

CHAPTER 18

BAUN SCORES ON ONE LEG

Hockey players are known for being the toughest of the tough. They will play through anything to win, especially if there is a championship on the line. When it comes to the Stanley Cup final, players would have to be missing a leg to not play.

That was almost the case in 1951 for Toronto Maple Leafs defenceman, Bobby Baun.

Baun was part of the Toronto Dynasty that would see the team win three straight Stanley Cups between 1963 and 1965 and then another surprise Cup in 1967. Although never an offensive threat — the most goals he ever scored in a season was eight — Baun was an important part of the Maple Leafs defense.

Despite finishing the season in third place, the Leafs and the fourth-place Detroit Red Wings would stun the Montreal Canadiens and Chicago Blackhawks in the first round of the playoffs. And even though they had finished ahead of the Red Wings, the Leafs were down three games to two as game six began at Detroit's Olympia Stadium.

The game went back and forth. Each time Detroit scored to take the lead, Toronto would come back and tie the game. With the game tied late in the third period, Baun blocked a shot, and the puck struck him on the ankle, and he fell to the ice in pain. He got up, but after the faceoff, he fell back on the ice. Unable to stand, he was taken off on a stretcher. Not long after, Gordie Howe would score to give Detroit the lead. But when Billy Harris tied the game late to send it to overtime, Baun knew what he had to do.

With doctors telling him otherwise, Baun insisted that his leg be taped up and frozen so he could return to the ice. When the overtime period started, Baun limped out onto the Leafs bench. He wouldn't have to wait long before he was on the ice.

With the puck in the Detroit end of the ice, Baun stopped a clearing attempt at the Red Wing's blueline and fired a shot at the net. Through a maze of players, the puck somehow went in, giving the Leafs a win and tying the series.

Inspired by his bravery, the Leafs cruised to a 4-0, game seven win and a third consecutive Cup win. A few days later, it was revealed that Baun had scored his famous goal and played in game seven with a broken leg.

"That's how important it was to win the Stanley Cup," he would later say.

Baun's demonstration of dedication to his team and that all-important Stanley Cup is a valuable lesson to learn. Of course, when you're injured, you should rest and recover, but perhaps we can learn metaphorically.

Setbacks are normal; they show up everywhere, but we should never let them hold us back from carrying on. Use setbacks as a learning opportunity–what went wrong, and how can you improve in the future?

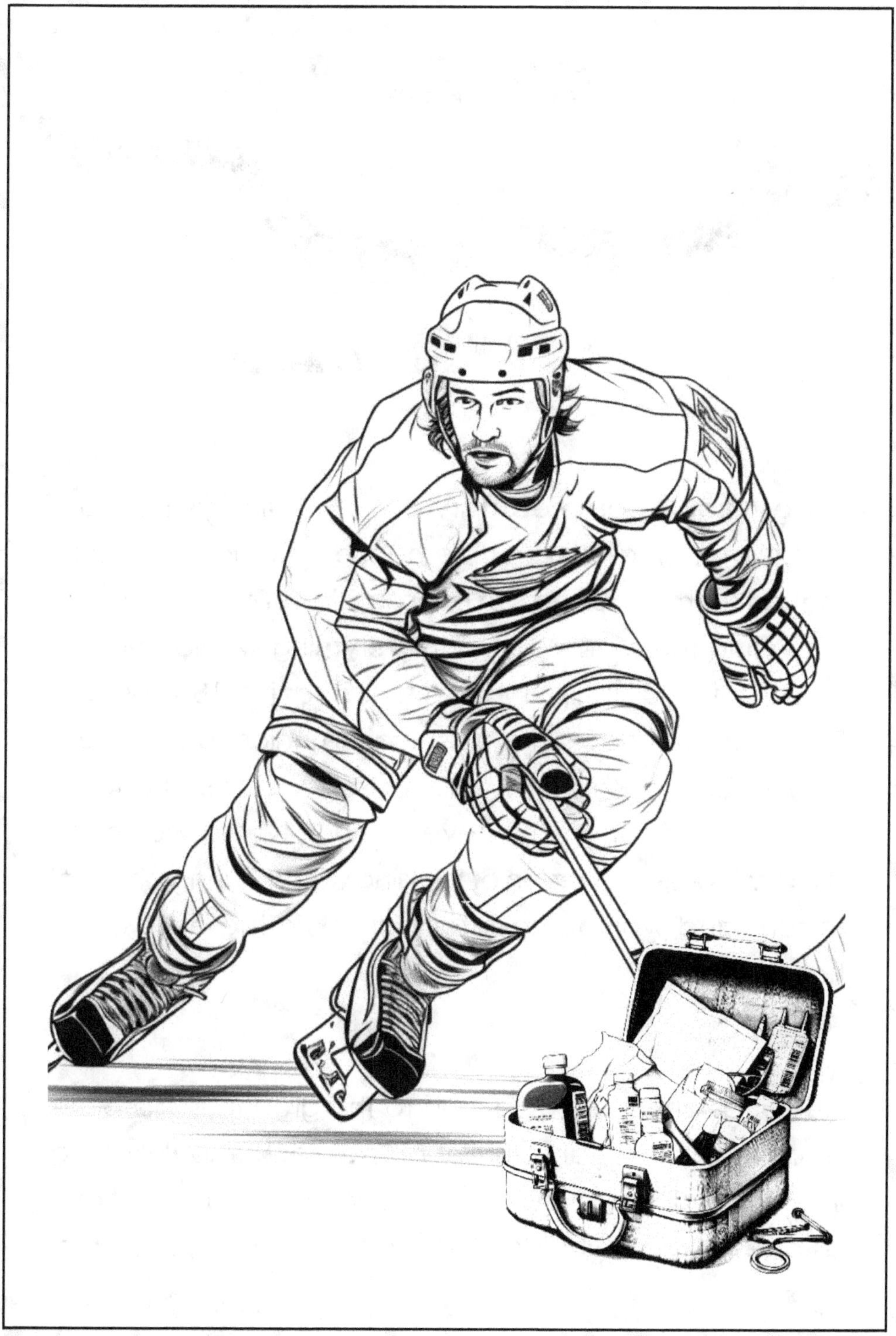

CHAPTER 19

ADJUST YOUR VISION

Greg Neeld, born February 25, 1955, always had big ambitions in the world of ice hockey. Neeld wanted to make it to the NHL and put every action in place in hopes of getting there one day. But everything would change on a fateful day in 1973 when Neeld was just 18 years old. During an Ontario Hockey Association junior game, Neeld played for the Toronto Marlboros against the Kitchener Rangers and suffered a severe injury. Neeld was high-sticked (hockey's version of tackling without using physical touch) and was accidentally struck in the eye with a hockey stick.

Neeld, as anyone would, falls to the ground in absolute agony, and the game is put on pause. Without getting into all the details, Neeld would end up losing his left eye as a result of this incident. He was, of course, in panic, thinking his career as a hockey player would be over before it even really began—he was crushed. Everyone thought he'd be the next Bobby Orr, but this sudden twist of fate looked like that would never be the case.

But Neeld, after recovering, knew that this could not be it for him—his journey was far from over. Unfortunately, despite desperate attempts to make it work, Neeld would not be able to play in the NHL. They had a rule requiring all players to have vision in both eyes. As much as various teams were passionately rooting for him, they just couldn't find a way to get around this rule.

Sure, there were a lot of setbacks that Neeld was facing because of his injury, but he still managed to achieve a lot. He would go on to play in the World Hockey Association (WHA) and the North American Hockey League (NAHL), as these leagues weren't picky about having a 20/20 vision. Over a 10-year period, Neeld played over 300 games in these other leagues and scored 84 goals. It's clear that, despite his unique situation, he was still able to achieve a lifelong dream. Neeld's injury led to a new rule in the Canadian Amateur Hockey Association, requiring all minor hockey players to wear facial protection on the field.

Neeld's injury teaches us that life comes with setbacks. In fact, setbacks are very normal. Sure, maybe we won't experience something as extreme as Neeld's, but we may experience similar setbacks. Maybe circumstances mean that you can't chase the same dream anymore. But let Neeld's be an inspiration—there is always another route.

Neeld also teaches us that, despite setbacks, he was able to continue having fun. So, when you face a similar obstacle and feel disheartened, remember that the root of playing sports is always having fun and making good memories.

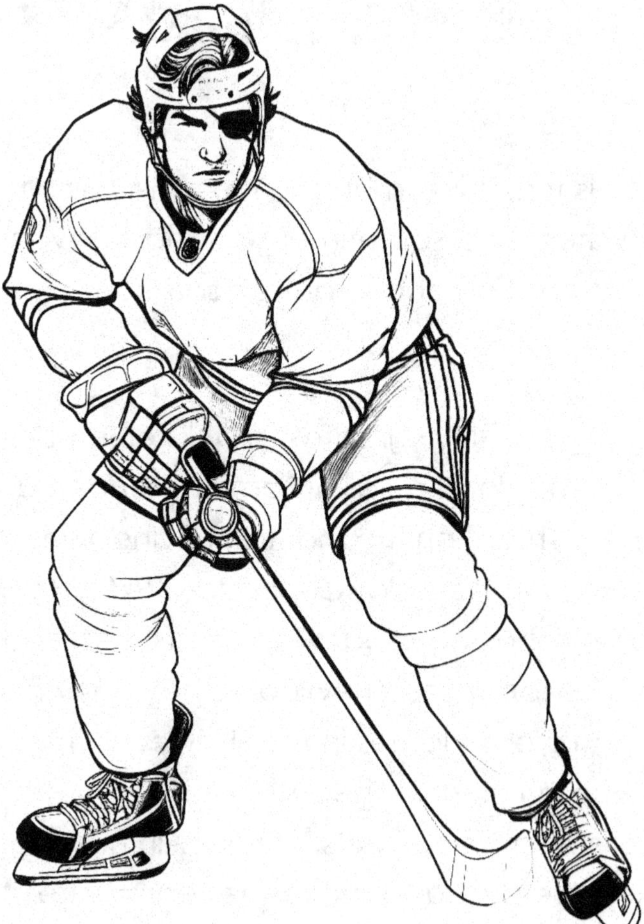

CHAPTER 20

THE MERRY PRANKSTER

Hockey is fun. It is fun on the ice, and it is fun with your teammates. And sometimes, it is made even more fun when you pull an epic prank on someone.

Possibly the all-time greatest prankster in hockey history was Guy Lapointe, a Hall of Fame defenceman and part of the 'Big Three' on the Montreal Canadiens teams that won four straight Stanley Cups in the 1970s. He was known for putting shaving cream in players' skates and shoes, moving a teammate's new car so he'd think it was stolen, putting player's clothes in the shower so they'd have to improvise a mix-matched silly outfit to get home, and even stealing his coach's whistle. All these lighthearted pranks were pulled to make the teams' stressful times a little more enjoyable.

But let's talk about one of his most famous pranks of all time, which was pulled on his Hall of Fame goaltender, Ken Dryden. Dryden was a highly intellectual member of the team who, along with being a goalie, was also a reputable lawyer (he'd go on to author several books and be a Member of Parliament in Canada). One night, after a team dinner, the restaurant brought out ice cream and chocolate sauce for the team's dessert. Lapointe had paid the waiters to bring a 'special' dessert for him, which they did. He then pretended he was too full to eat and offered the dessert to Dryden, who accepted—I mean, who wouldn't accept a free dessert? Little did Dryden know the ice cream was, in fact, not actually ice cream. Turns out, it was actually sour cream, so it was quite the shock when Dryden took a big scoop. The awful sour taste exploded in Dryden's mouth, but he found it hilarious. Want to know what's even funnier? This was Dryden's first proper introduction to Lapointe, and, oh, what a mark he left on the goaltender.

After all, what are friends and defensemen for?

This crafty prankster teaches us that having fun is so important. Sometimes, situations like the NHL can be stressful and overwhelming. Throwing in a bit of lighthearted fun can make it more bearable and take that pressure away.

So, when you find yourself in a stressful situation or see your friend seems overwhelmed, maybe try finding a way to make fun of the situation. I mean, it worked for Lapointe, right?

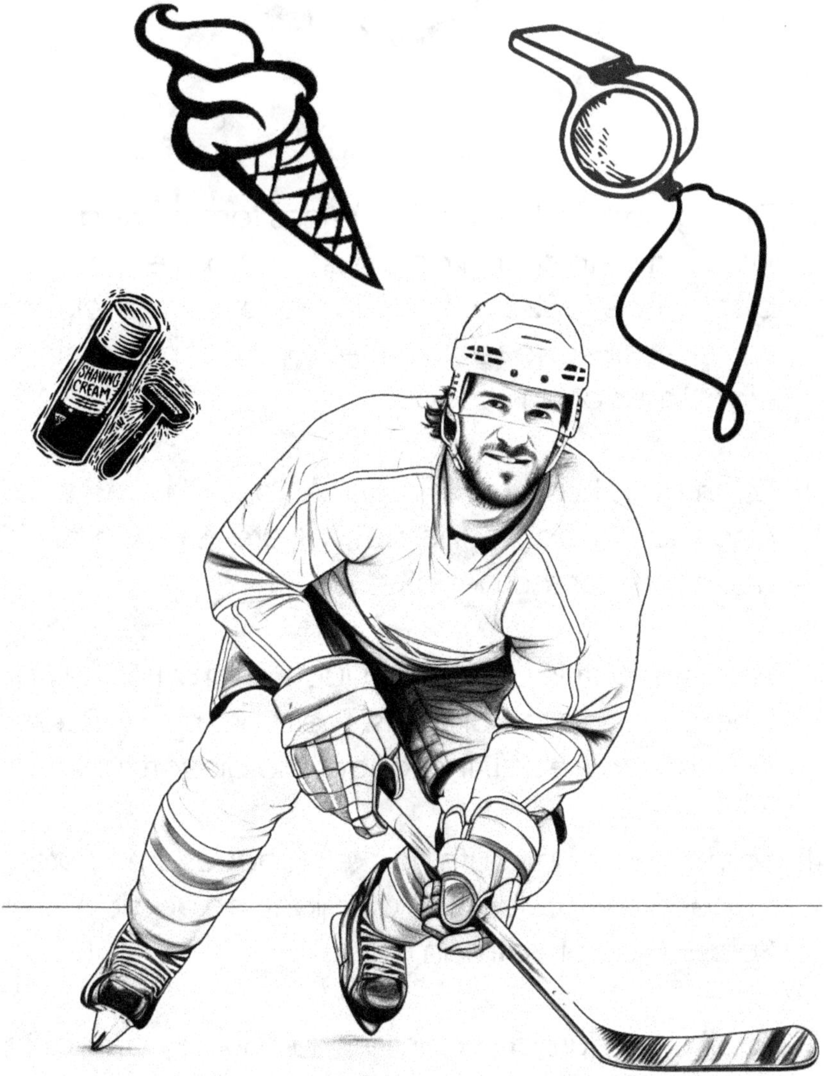

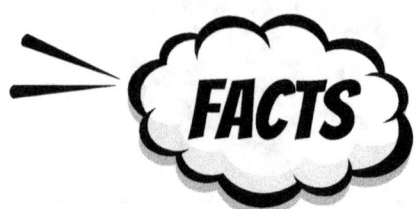

1. During games, Detroit Red Wings fans have a strange tradition of throwing octopuses onto the ice. It dates back to the 1952 Stanley Cup playoffs, when eight wins were required to secure the trophy, representing the eight limbs of an octopus.

2. Each sport has its own lingo. A "biscuit in the basket" refers to a puck in the net, whereas a "sin bin" is a nickname for the penalty box.

3. As a superstition for good luck, many players grow beards during the playoffs. The more magnificent the postseason beard, the longer the playoff run.

4. Some goalies in youth hockey leagues like to dress up in superhero costumes. You might see goalies wearing Spider-Man or Batman masks!

5. Tooth loss during a game is surprisingly prevalent in hockey. Some players have unusual customs, such as throwing their missing teeth into the crowd or using them to make jewelry.

CONCLUSION

And there you have it—how inspiring are these athletes? Despite challenges, they rose to the occasion and overcame.

Guy Lapointe taught us that lighthearted humor and funny pranks are some of the best ways to bond with your team, making stressful situations a little more fun. An unexpected spooky bat demonstrated how disappointing games and bad weather can be improved with the tiniest influence of eerie nature. And what about Tyler Motte? He showed us that opening up about our mental health struggles is just as important as getting help for our physical health.

So, what's next for you? Yes, you! You, who's reading this right now. Think about these short stories—what was your favorite one? Who inspired you the most? What have you personally learned from these inspiring athletes? Whether it's overcoming those who underestimate you or finding alternative routes to achieve your dreams, I hope it's something valuable.